Handbook for Clinical Trials of Imaging and Image-Guided Interventions

T0176947

Handbook for Clinical Trials of Imaging and Image-Guided Interventions

EDITED BY

Nancy A. Obuchowski, PhD

Vice Chair for Quantitative Health Sciences,
Cleveland Clinic Foundation, and
Professor of Medicine at the Cleveland Clinic Lerner College of
Medicine of Case Western Reserve University, USA

and

G. Scott Gazelle, MD, MPH, PhD, FACR

Director Emeritus of the Massachusetts General Hospital
Institute for Technology Assessment,
Professor of Radiology at Harvard Medical School, and
Professor in the Department of Health Policy and Management
at the Harvard School of Public Health, USA

WILEY Blackwell

Published by John Wiley & Sons, Inc., Hoboken, New Jersey

Published simultaneously in Canada

For general information on our other products and services or for technical support, please contact our Customer Care Department within the United States at (800) 762-2974, outside the United States at (317) 572-3993 or fax (317) 572-4002.

Wiley also publishes its books in a variety of electronic formats. Some content that appears in print may not be available in electronic formats. For more information about Wiley products, visit our web site at www.wiley.com.

Library of Congress Cataloging-in-Publication Data:

Names: Obuchowski, Nancy A., editor. | Gazelle, G. Scott., editor.
Title: Handbook for clinical trials of imaging and image-guided interventions / edited by Nancy A. Obuchowski and G. Scott Gazelle.
Description: Hoboken, New Jersey : John Wiley & Sons, Inc., [2016] | Includes bibliographical references and index.
Identifiers: LCCN 2015038320 | ISBN 9781118849750 (pbk.)
Subjects: | MESH: Clinical Trials as Topic. | Diagnostic Imaging. | Radiotherapy. | Surgery, Computer-Assisted.
Classification: LCC RC78.7.D53 | NLM WN 180 | DDC 616.07/54–dc23
LC record available at http://lccn.loc.gov/2015038320

Cover image: Background image X-ray of a fracture of an upper arm © Thomas Hacker/gettyimages

Printed and bound in Malaysia by Vivar Printing Sdn Bhd

1 2016

Contents

Contributors

Elizabeth C. Adami, BS
Department of Radiology, Massachusetts General Hospital & Harvard Medical School, Boston, MA, USA

Todd A. Alonzo, PHD
Department of Preventive Medicine, University of Southern California, Los Angeles, CA, USA

Jeffrey D. Blume, PHD
Department of Biostatistics, Vanderbilt University, Nashville, TN, USA

Ruth C. Carlos, MD, MS
Department of Radiology, University of Michigan Institute for Health Policy and Innovation and the Program for Imaging Comparative Effectiveness and Health Services Research, Ann Arbor, MI, USA

Gary S. Dorfman, MD
Department of Radiology, Weill Cornell Medical College, New York, NY, USA

G. Scott Gazelle, MD, MPH, PHD
Massachusetts General Hospital & Harvard Medical School, Boston, MA, USA

Stephen M. Hahn, MD
The University of Texas MD Anderson Cancer Center, Houston, TX, USA

Udo Hoffmann, MD, MPH
Department of Radiology, Massachusetts General Hospital & Harvard Medical School, Boston, MA, USA

Sayeh Lavasani, MD, MSC
Department of Oncology, Barbara Ann Karmanos Cancer Institute, Wayne State University, Detroit, MI, USA

Janie M. Lee, MD, MSC
Department of Radiology, University of Washington, Boston, MA, USA

Constance D. Lehman, MD, PHD
Department of Radiology, University of Washington; Department of Radiology, Massachusetts General Hospital, Boston, MA, USA

Michael T. Lu, MD
Department of Radiology, Massachusetts General Hospital & Harvard Medical School, Boston, MA, USA

Ali Mahinbakht, MD, MSc
Barbara Ann Karmanos Cancer Institute, Wayne State University, Detroit, MI, USA; University of Liverpool, Liverpool, UK

David A. Mankoff, MD, PHD
Department of Radiology, Perelman School of Medicine, University of Pennsylvania, Philadelphia, PA, USA

Diana L. Miglioretti, PHD
Department of Public Health Sciences, University of California Davis School of Medicine, Davis, CA, USA

Nancy A. Obuchowski, PHD
Quantitative Health Sciences, Cleveland Clinic Foundation, Cleveland, OH, USA

Pari V. Pandharipande, MD, MPH
Massachusetts General Hospital & Harvard Medical School, Boston, MA, USA

Anthony F. Shields, MD, PHD
Department of Oncology, Barbara Ann Karmanos Cancer Institute, Wayne State University, Detroit, MI, USA

Alicia Y. Toledano, SCD
Biostatistics Consulting, LLC, Kensington, MD, USA

CHAPTER 1

Imaging technology assessment

Pari V. Pandharipande and G. Scott Gazelle

Massachusetts General Hospital & Harvard Medical School, Boston, MA, USA

KEY POINTS

- The ability to define the most appropriate roles for imaging and imaging-guided interventions in medical care will be a critical goal for the future success of radiology; as such, ways to overcome current barriers to successful technology assessments must be a priority.

- A six-level hierarchical model of technology assessments, focused in diagnostic testing, provides a useful framework for understanding how research concerning a technology's worth can progress from assessments of its technical efficacy to those of its societal value.

- Randomized controlled trials in imaging are commonly not feasible; alternative research methods (e.g., observational studies leveraging large data repositories) can provide practical solutions to addressing this problem.

- In order to benefit patients most in the broader context of healthcare, all technology assessments should be initiated with an eye toward future studies that will test the technology's worth at the societal level.

The continued success of radiology, as a discipline that can contribute meaningfully to the care of patients and improvements in public health, will depend upon our ability to define the most appropriate roles for imaging in modern medical care. In the past three decades, there have been astounding advances in imaging technologies; in parallel, utilization has increased rapidly [1–3]. Despite quick dissemination of such technologies into practice, the value that they add to patient care, in many instances, has yet to be clearly established [1–3]. Three barriers to related research efforts merit specific mention [2–4]. First, because imaging technologies typically address intermediate steps in a patient's care, it can be extremely difficult to conduct studies that reliably link imaging results to patient outcomes. Second, imaging technologies evolve rapidly, which frequently obviates the relevance of studies focusing on long-term patient outcomes. Third, there are few investigators who are adequately trained to conduct rigorous

---

Handbook for Clinical Trials of Imaging and Image-Guided Interventions, First Edition.
Edited by Nancy A. Obuchowski and G. Scott Gazelle.
© 2016 John Wiley & Sons, Inc. Published 2016 by John Wiley & Sons, Inc.

assessments of imaging and image-guided interventions—until now, research focusing on technology development has had a greater priority. In the current era of healthcare reform, however, the value of healthcare is viewed increasingly through the lens of patient outcomes and societal costs, and efforts to overcome the barriers described earlier have emerged as a priority [2–5]. In this chapter, we first provide an overview of the different levels of evidence that define technology assessments in imaging [6–10]. We then introduce three case examples; together, they highlight common approaches and challenges to technology assessments in imaging and serve as a platform for discussing key research topics that will be covered in this book.

1.1 Six levels of evidence: a model of technology assessments in imaging

Models that are commonly used to categorize evidence in medicine do not translate well to diagnostic imaging, because they are typically centered on therapy rather than diagnosis. Since the 1970s, pioneers in technology assessment and imaging have contributed to the development and refinement of a six-level hierarchical model that is specific to diagnostic technologies [6–9]. The levels include (i) technical efficacy, (ii) diagnostic accuracy, (iii) impact on diagnostic thinking, (iv) impact on therapeutic planning, (v) impact on patient outcomes, and (vi) impact on societal outcomes [2, 6–10]. The model is hierarchical with respect to the scope of the evidence's impact: its spectrum "begins" with technical efficacy (*Level 1*) and "ends" with societal outcomes (*Level 6*). The model is also hierarchical with respect to the potential of a technology's impact: it implies, for example, that a given technology needs to demonstrate a certain level of diagnostic accuracy (*Level 2*) in order to produce favorable health and economic outcomes at the societal level (*Level 6*). However, a technology's success at one level does not necessarily predict its success at higher levels; for example, a highly accurate technology may not meaningfully—or positively—affect patient outcomes [6, 11]. Each level and the types of research appropriate to evaluate efficacy at that level are described below.

1.1.1 Level 1: technical efficacy
Technical efficacy is judged by measurements that pertain to image generation (in diagnostic imaging) and procedural feasibility (in interventional radiology) [6, 7, 11]. These measurements are preclinical; they serve as the basis for continual, iterative improvements until the technology is ready for testing and use in clinical practice [6, 7, 11]. Commonly applied metrics may include spatial and contrast resolution (for diagnostic techniques) and the precision of catheter, needle, or probe localization (for interventional techniques). A review of technical efficacy

parameters is commonly required by regulatory authorities—such as the US Food and Drug Administration—prior to a technology's dissemination into practice.

1.1.2 Level 2: diagnostic accuracy

Diagnostic accuracy is judged by multiple metrics of test performance. Here, we will discuss the three most common: (i) sensitivity and specificity, (ii) positive and negative predictive value (PPV and NPV, respectively), and (iii) receiver-operating characteristic (ROC) curves [11–14]. Each reflects a different window into the ability of a technology to detect disease. Sensitivity and specificity reflect a technology's ability to detect true positive (among disease-positive) cases and true negative (among disease-negative) cases within a study population. PPV and NPV also reflect the technology's ability to detect true positive and true negative cases but instead among *test positive* and *test negative* cases, respectively. Therefore, PPV and NPV—unlike sensitivity and specificity—depend heavily on disease prevalence within the study population. As a result, study-derived estimates of PPV and NPV are specific to populations with similar disease prevalence as the study population.

ROC curves, which plot sensitivity (*y*-axis) against 1-specificity (*x*-axis), provide insight into the trade-offs that occur when using different thresholds for calling a test "positive" [11, 13, 14]. When studies include data from multiple readers and/or multiple sites of care, a summary ROC curve may be generated, providing insights into the capabilities and limitations of an imaging technology that are more generalizable. (See Chapter 9 for a detailed discussion of ROC curves.)

Research evaluating the diagnostic accuracy of imaging technologies is frequently challenged by the identification of a suitable reference standard. Here, we highlight three common predicaments [11]; further details can be found in Chapter 7. First, in certain circumstances, an imaging test result may be less likely to be verified (e.g., undergo follow-up biopsy) than others. This can occur, for example, when a positive imaging test is typically verified in routine care, but negative or indeterminate results are not. In such situations, the resulting "verification bias" could distort corresponding estimates of test performance. Second, imaging technologies sometimes can detect more underlying pathology than a commonly accepted reference standard. Consider, for example, a patient who undergoes a liver biopsy for the detection of hepatic steatosis. The biopsy (reference standard) may be falsely negative, due to sampling of an unaffected area of the liver; however, imaging of the whole liver may more accurately reveal patchy areas of fatty infiltration throughout the liver. Using such a reference standard (a so-called tarnished gold standard) can result in inappropriately low estimates of sensitivity and specificity. Third, in many scenarios, the only reasonable reference standard is patient outcomes based on long-term follow-up, for example, disease progression or regression. Given the large number of additional tests and treatments that an individual may experience during follow-up, it can be very difficult to attribute long-term outcomes to the results of a given imaging test. When defining a reference standard in a study of diagnostic accuracy, investigators typically must address one or more of the mentioned obstacles or, at minimum, understand how such obstacles may affect their results.

1.1.3 Levels 3 and 4: impact on diagnostic thinking and therapeutic planning

The impact of imaging technologies on diagnostic thinking (Level 3) is generally assessed by determining changes in physicians' diagnoses and/or their diagnostic confidence following the performance of an imaging study [2, 6, 7, 10, 15–17]. Moving progressively "closer" to patient outcomes, Level 4 studies measure the impact of imaging technologies on therapeutic planning (Level 4) by judging a technology's effect on patient management [2, 6, 7, 10, 15, 16]. The principal challenge in obtaining such measurements is knowing what would have happened, under real clinical conditions, had the imaging test not been performed. To determine this, hypothetical questions are generally posed to physicians, such as, *"what would you have done if this imaging test were unavailable?"* [15, 16]. These hypothetical questions are known to be cognitively burdensome and subject to various biases; nevertheless, they can also provide information that is critically important for assessing the value of new imaging technologies. The National Oncologic PET Registry (NOPR) provides one of the best examples of how this information can be requested, reported, and used to gain insight into the projected value of a new imaging technology [18, 19].

1.1.4 Level 5: patient outcomes

Patient outcomes that are associated with imaging can be evaluated with a wide spectrum of measures [2–5]. Metrics may address short- or immediate-term outcomes (e.g., rates of allergic reactions, complications, or postprocedural mortality) or long-term outcomes (e.g., rates of overall survival, disease-specific survival, progression-free survival, or life expectancy and quality of life). As mentioned, patient-level outcomes are difficult to measure in a way that can be confidently attributed to imaging. To reliably measure patient outcomes associated with imaging, randomized controlled trials (RCTs) are typically needed. In such studies, patients are randomized, for example, to undergo an imaging technology under investigation versus the standard of care [20–23]. Because differences in outcomes between the study groups are commonly small, large sample sizes are often required to achieve adequate power. This, combined with the need to conduct long-term follow-up, can make imaging-related RCTs prohibitively expensive. Nevertheless, when a substantial proportion of the population may be affected, the information yielded may justify such costs; the National Lung Screening Trial [20] exemplifies one such circumstance among several [20–23].

Additional study designs permit outcomes evaluations and, in many cases, may represent a more practical and feasible approach. Two merit specific mention. First, **population-level observational studies** that leverage "big data"—for example, data repositories or registries that are large enough to require specialized programming and analytics for their analysis—may provide a new window into imaging-related outcomes [4]. While such research is still subject to typical biases of observational studies, it may offer new opportunities to evaluate relationships between imaging technologies and patient outcomes, particularly in settings where such analyses were not previously feasible due to limitations of study power. Second, "pragmatic" trial designs are gaining traction, though they are in their infancy as an outcomes research method [4, 24]. **Pragmatic trials** are those that attempt to deliver a low-burden intervention to a wide variety of practice settings, with less restrictive inclusion criteria as compared to typical RCTs [4, 24]. Data collection is typically passive, occurring, for example, through automated collection of specific outcomes that are already recorded in participating centers' electronic medical record systems [4]. The primary advantage of pragmatic trials over traditional RCTs is their greater generalizability to "real-world" settings; the primary disadvantage is that because of their less stringent study designs, they are more vulnerable to bias [4, 24].

1.1.5 Level 6: societal efficacy

Societal efficacy is judged by whether an imaging technology represents a good use of societal resources. By definition, societal efficacy must account for both health outcomes (clinical effectiveness) and economic outcomes (costs) associated with the use of an imaging modality [25–27]. Ideally, costs and effectiveness should be evaluated using a societal perspective and a lifetime horizon [25–27]. Using a societal perspective to estimate costs is important because resource allocation decisions are often made at the societal level. Using a lifetime horizon for estimating costs and effectiveness is also important because in many circumstances, the risks, benefits, and costs of imaging technologies are strongly influenced by the downstream care pathways that occur as a result of the imaging test result(s). Put another way, the health and economic outcomes associated with subsequent care, rather than the imaging technology itself, strongly influence the value of imaging. Most analyses of societal efficacy employ cost-effectiveness analysis, adhering closely to the guidelines put forth by the Panel on Cost-Effectiveness in Health and Medicine, convened in the 1990s by the US Public Health Service [25–27].

In the United States, a consistent challenge of cost-effectiveness analysis, from the standpoint of policymakers, pertains to the interpretation of results [28–30]. In a standard cost-effectiveness analysis, the primary results are expressed in terms of one or more incremental cost-effectiveness ratios (ICERs) that are associated with corresponding diagnostic testing and/or treatment options. An ICER represents the additional cost required to achieve an additional unit of outcome (commonly life-years or quality-adjusted life-years). In theory, whether or not a technology is an efficient use of resources is judged by comparing such ICERs to a societal willingness-to-pay (WTP) threshold, which represents the price that a society is willing to pay to increase life expectancy (or quality-adjusted life expectancy) in a target population [25–27]. In the United States, there is no "hard" threshold beyond which a technology is considered too expensive, a circumstance that often challenges the interpretation of ICERs resulting from cost-effectiveness analyses [28–30]. Recently, a $100,000–$150,000 WTP threshold has been suggested as a guideline for US analyses, but this value will undoubtedly be subject to debate and revision in future years, to account for inflation and an evolving economic and healthcare climate [30]. See Chapter 11 for further details.

1.2 Case examples: introducing technology assessment methods into study design

Technology assessments that correspond to each of the described levels of evidence present investigators with common challenges, several of which have been discussed earlier. As in any discipline, however, the best way to know and anticipate such challenges is to gain experience in doing the research itself. In lieu of this—as a proxy—it is worthwhile to think through the design of typical assessments of imaging technologies. Drawing from the principles presented earlier, we introduce three hypothetical areas of research inquiry, selected to span both diagnostic and interventional imaging technologies. The examples illustrate how technology assessment research methods may be applied in a variety of clinical settings and serve as a platform for discussions throughout the remainder of this book.

Case example 1.1 A New Liver Blood-Pool Agent for Detecting Colorectal Metastases at CT: Evaluation of Diagnostic Accuracy

Unlike in many other cancer settings, isolated liver metastases in patients with colorectal cancer may be treated for cure [31]. As a result, accurate detection of liver metastases from colorectal cancer is an important component of treatment planning in these patients. Suppose that a hypothetical blood-pool agent ("Agent A") is developed specifically for the identification of colorectal metastases in the liver at CT and that its safety in human subjects has been established. Whether or not Agent A is superior in detecting liver metastases, relative to the current standard of care (e.g., CT with Agent B), is unknown. Readers may consider what types of study designs could *(i) determine whether Agent A can more accurately identify liver metastases than Agent B, (ii) identify appropriate thresholds for positivity when using Agent A (vs. Agent B) as a CT contrast agent, and (iii) determine whether the use of Agent A can result in improved patient outcomes or more efficient use of societal resources than the current standard of care.*

Case example 1.2 A New Biologic for Metastatic Breast Cancer: Evaluation of Treatment Response with ¹⁸F-FDG-PET Imaging

Consider a new type of drug—Biologic A—that is found to be highly effective in the treatment of a subset (20%) of patients with metastatic breast cancer. Unfortunately, no test is available that allows for *a priori* determination of whether a given patient will respond. Biologic A carries a small risk (1% per year) of death from severe immunosuppression, and its cost exceeds $100,000 per month. As a result, there is substantial interest in identifying patients, as early as possible in the course of their therapy, who are likely to be responders. At ¹⁸F-FDG-PET imaging, uptake of ¹⁸F-FDG correlates with tumor viability, and decreased uptake following treatment generally correlates with tumor responsiveness, but the thresholds for uptake in separating respondents from nonrespondents are imperfect. Moreover, some individuals declare themselves as respondents 1–2 months later than others. Readers may consider what types of study designs could *(i) determine the extent to which FDG-PET is capable of distinguishing responders from nonresponders and (ii) identify optimal thresholds—guided by patient outcomes—for distinguishing these populations.*

Case example 1.3 Minimally Invasive Therapies for Early Lung Cancer: A Comparison of Imaging-Guided Radiofrequency Ablation versus Stereotactic Ablative Radiotherapy

In certain situations, early lung cancers may be identified in patients who cannot undergo surgery, for example, due to advanced age or multiple comorbidities. In these circumstances, minimally invasive approaches may offer an opportunity for treatment and cure. An increasing number of options are available [32–34]. In one option, imaging-guided radiofrequency ablation (RFA), a radiologist inserts a probe into the tumor under imaging guidance and then delivers radiofrequency energy to "kill" tumor cells [32, 33]. In another option, stereotactic ablative radiotherapy (SABR), a radiation oncologist delivers a highly localized, therapeutic radiation dose to treat the tumor [34]. Each option has different risks and benefits and a different profile of complications. Readers may consider what types of study designs could *(i) determine and compare the clinical efficacy of each treatment, (ii) measure and compare quality of life associated with each treatment, and (iii) determine the relative cost-effectiveness of the different treatments.*

1.3 Conclusion

In this chapter, we have provided a broad introduction to the assessment of imaging technologies, reviewing a six-level hierarchical model for categorizing evidence in diagnostic imaging [6–9]. In addition, we have provided hypothetical areas of research inquiry, to set the stage for further discussions of research design and methods in subsequent chapters (e.g., ROC curves, survival estimates, quality-of-life evaluation, etc.). When considering the hierarchy and the clinical examples presented, our primary take-home point is the following: while robust studies of an imaging technology's technical efficacy and diagnostic accuracy are important, they are insufficient in demonstrating the technology's value to patients. In order to benefit patients most in the broader context of healthcare, technology assessments—*at all levels*—should be initiated with an eye toward future studies that will test the technology's worth at the societal level.

References

1 Smith-Bindman, R., D.L. Miglioretti, and E.B. Larson, Rising Use Of Diagnostic Medical Imaging In A Large Integrated Health System. *Health Aff*, 2008. **27**(6): p. 1491–1502.
2 Gazelle, G.S., et al., A framework for assessing the value of diagnostic imaging in the era of comparative effectiveness research. *Radiology*, 2011. **261**(3): p. 692–698.
3 Pandharipande, P.V. and G.S. Gazelle, Comparative effectiveness research: what it means for radiology. *Radiology*, 2009. **253**(3): p. 600–605.
4 Lee, C.I. and J.G. Jarvik, Patient-centered outcomes research in radiology: trends in funding and methodology. *Acad Radiol*, 2014. **21**(9): p. 1156–1161.
5 Carlos, R.C., et al., Patient-centered outcomes in imaging: quantifying value. *J Am Coll Radiol*, 2012. **9**(10): p. 725–728.
6 Fryback, D.G. and J.R. Thornbury, The efficacy of diagnostic imaging. *Med Decis Making*, 1991. **11**(2): p. 88–94.
7 Thornbury, J.R., Eugene W. Caldwell Lecture. Clinical efficacy of diagnostic imaging: love it or leave it. *AJR Am J Roentgenol*, 1994. **162**(1): p. 1–8.
8 Fineberg, H.V., Evaluation of computed tomography: achievement and challenge. *AJR Am J Roentgenol*, 1978. **131**(1): p. 1–4.
9 Fineberg, H.V., R. Bauman, and M. Sosman, Computerized cranial tomography. Effect on diagnostic and therapeutic plans. *JAMA*, 1977. **238**(3): p. 224–227.
10 Pearson, S.D., et al., Assessing the comparative effectiveness of a diagnostic technology: CT colonography. *Health AFF (Millwood)*, 2008. **2008**(27): p. 6.
11 Gazelle, G.S., Cost-Effectiveness of Imaging and Surgery in Patients with Colorectal Cancer Liver Metastases. 1999, Harvard University, U.S. Copyright # TX 4-973-835.
12 McNeil, B.J. and S.J.Adelstein, Determining the value of diagnostic and screening tests. *J Nucl Med*, 1976. **17**(6): p. 439–448.
13 Goodenough, D.J., K. Rossmann, and L.B. Lusted, Radiographic applications of receiver operating characteristic (ROC) curves. *Radiology*, 1974. **110**(1): p. 89–95.
14 McNeil, B.J. and J.A. Hanley, Statistical approaches to the analysis of receiver operating characteristic (ROC) curves. *Med Decis Making*, 1984. **4**(2): p. 137–150.
15 Abujudeh, H.H., R. Kaewlai, and P.M. McMahon, Abdominopelvic CT increases diagnostic certainty and guides management decisions: a prospective investigation of 584 patients in a large academic medical center. *AJR Am J Roentgenol*, 2011. **196**(2): p. 238–242.
16 Esses, D., Birnbaum, A., Bijur, P., Shah, S., Gleyzer, A., Gallagher, E.J., Ability of CT to alter decision making in elderly patients with acute abdominal pain. *Am J Emerg Med*, 2004. **22**(4): p. 270–272.
17 Nagurney, J.T., Brown, D.F., Chang, Y., Sane, S, Wang, A.C., Weiner, J.B., Use of diagnostic testing in the emergency department for patients presenting with non-traumatic abdominal pain. *J Emerg Med*, 2003. **25**(4): p. 363–371.
18 Hillner, B.E., et al., The National Oncologic PET Registry (NOPR): design and analysis plan. *J Nucl Med*, 2007. **48**(11): p. 1901–1908.
19 Aberle, D.R., et al., Reduced lung-cancer mortality with low-dose computed tomographic screening. *N Engl J Med*, 2011. **365**(5): p. 395–409.

20 Jarvik, J.G., et al., Rapid magnetic resonance imaging vs radiographs for patients with low back pain: a randomized controlled trial. *JAMA*, 2003. **289**(21): p. 2810–2818.
21 Hillner, B.E., et al., Impact of positron emission tomography/computed tomography and positron emission tomography (PET) alone on expected management of patients with cancer: initial results from the National Oncologic PET Registry. *J Clin Oncol*, 2008. **26**(13): p. 2155–2161.
22 Smith-Bindman, R., et al., Ultrasonography versus computed tomography for suspected nephrolithiasis. *N Engl J Med*, 2014. **371**(12): p. 1100–1110.
23 Hoffman, U., et al., Coronary CT angiography versus standard evaluation in acute chest pain. *N Engl J Med*, 2012. **367**(4): p. 299–308.
24 Lurie, J.D. and T.S. Morgan, Pros and cons of pragmatic clinical trials. *J Comp Eff Res*, 2013. **2**(1): p. 53–58.
25 Hunink, M.G., Outcomes research and cost-effectiveness analysis in radiology. *Eur Radiol*, 1996. **6**(5): p. 615–620.
26 Weinstein, M.C., et al., Recommendations of the Panel on Cost-effectiveness in Health and Medicine. *JAMA*, 1996. **276**(15): p. 1253–1258.
27 Gazelle, G.S., et al., Cost-effectiveness analysis in the assessment of diagnostic imaging technologies. *Radiology*, 2005. **235**(2): p. 361–370.
28 Winkelmayer, W.C., et al., Health economic evaluations: the special case of end-stage renal disease treatment. *Med Decis Making*, 2002. **22**(5): p. 417–430.
29 Neumann, P.J. and M.C. Weinstein, Legislating against use of cost-effectiveness information. *N Engl J Med*, 2010. **363**(16): p. 1495–1497.
30 Neumann, P.J., J.T. Cohen, and M.C. Weinstein, Updating cost-effectiveness—the curious resilience of the $50,000-per-QALY threshold. *N Engl J Med*, 2014. **371**(9): p. 796–797.
31 Chan, K.M., et al., Outcomes of resection for colorectal cancer hepatic metastases stratified by evolving eras of treatment. *World J Surg Oncol*, 2011. **9**: p. 174.
32 de Baere, T., G. Farouil, and F. Deschamps, Lung cancer ablation: what is the evidence? *Semin Interv Radiol*, 2013. **30**(2): p. 151–156.
33 Ridge C.A., S.B.Solomon, and R.H.Thornton, Thermal ablation of stage I non-small cell lung carcinoma. *Semin Interv Radiol*, 2014. **31**(2): p. 118–124.
34 Padda, S.K., et al., Early-stage non-small cell Lung cancer: surgery, stereotactic radiosurgery, and individualized adjuvant therapy. *Semin Oncol*, 2014. **41**(1): p. 40–56.

CHAPTER 2

Clinical trials of therapy

Sayeh Lavasani[1], Anthony F. Shields[1] and Ali Mahinbakht[1,2]

[1] *Barbara Ann Karmanos Cancer Institute, Wayne State University, Detroit, MI, USA*
[2] *University of Liverpool, Liverpool, UK*

KEY POINTS

- Clinical trials evolve from phase I to evaluate toxicity and early evidence of efficacy to comparative trials in phase III.

- The stated primary objective of a trial should be specific, simple, and of clinical importance since it will determine the success of the study and drive the sample size calculations.

- To select patients for these early trials, the investigator needs to carefully write the eligibility criteria to include a group of subjects that will result in generalizable information, but does not eliminate appropriate patients and impair accrual.

- The schedule for evaluation and treatment in trials needs to be practical to ensure accrual and minimize protocol deviations.

2.1 Phases I, II, and III: their goals and rationale

What is meant by a "clinical trial"? Clinical trials are any form of planned, prospective experiment that involves patients or healthy volunteers; they are designed to determine the utility of a diagnostic or imaging test or the efficacy and safety of a treatment. Clinical trials have different phases defined by the Food and Drug Administration (FDA); each phase has a different goal:

- **Phase 0**: Phase 0 is not routinely performed but is a microdosing study in a small group of subjects (10–15 individuals) to collect information on an agent's pharmacodynamics and pharmacokinetics. This phase does not give any data about the safety and efficacy of a therapy but helps to make a go/no-go decision [1]. Studies of the utility and safety of radionuclide imaging agents, which are used at tracer levels, may be considered phase 0 trials, while some may consider these phase I studies.

- **Phase I**: In phase I, safety is the primary concern, not efficacy. A phase I study is intended to identify a safe dose range. There is no control group in a phase

Handbook for Clinical Trials of Imaging and Image-Guided Interventions, First Edition.
Edited by Nancy A. Obuchowski and G. Scott Gazelle.

I study, and it is not randomized. There are generally a small number of subjects (usually between 20 and 80) [2]. Participants are healthy volunteers or seriously ill patients who have failed to respond to treatments [3]. The role of phase I trials in cancer trials has changed over the last few years. They often contain expansion cohorts of a particular cancer with a specific histology or genetic marker; these may at times substitute for more classic phase II trials to evaluate efficacy. Phase I trials may also include cohorts to assess different schedules, food effects for oral agents, and interactions with common supportive medications (e.g., acetaminophen). Such cohorts are sometimes added even after phase III trials have been performed and FDA licensing of the agent.

• **Phase II**: Phase II provides information about efficacy and also continues to investigate toxicity. Phase II trials may be randomized with a control arm of standard treatment or include multiple experimental arms. Phase II could be a screening trial for finding a few genuine medications from a large number of inactive and toxic drugs. Sample size is usually between a couple of dozen to a few hundred subjects [2]. Without a phase II trial, the chance of success in a phase III trial is very low.

• **Phase III**: When a new intervention is shown to be effective, it is necessary to compare it to the standard treatment in a large trial. Phase III is a randomized trial to assess the effectiveness of a new medication or intervention. In a phase III trial, investigators recruit a much larger number of subjects than in phase II. When working to assess small differences in efficacy between two interventions, thousands of subjects may be required. Despite promising results in phase II trials, phase III trials often show less efficacy (Figure 2.1) [4].

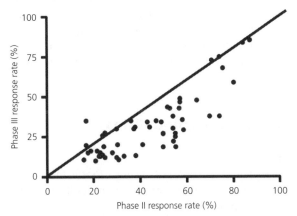

Figure 2.1 Comparison of response rates from phase II and phase III trials, redrawn. Source: Adapted from Zia [4].

- **Phase IV**: Phase IV is a postmarketing surveillance study after FDA approval. Phases I, II, and III are too small to identify rare but serious adverse effects. In addition, a phase IV study could detect long-term side effects of new interventions. Some harmful findings in phase IV could result in restrictions or stopping the sale of a drug. An example is rofecoxib.

2.2 Therapeutic roles: prevention, cure, and palliation

Clinical trials vary according to their goals. Clinical *therapeutic studies* investigate the effectiveness of a new treatment, which could be a new drug or a combination of existing drugs, radiation, new surgery, or immunotherapy.

A *prevention trial* assesses an intervention that could decrease the risk of a certain disease or reduce the recurrence rate. There are three levels of prevention: primary, secondary, and tertiary prevention. In primary prevention, there is no disease and the goal is to remove the cause. An example of primary prevention is vaccination. An example of secondary prevention is a mammogram to detect an early disease at an asymptomatic stage; therefore, it is a screening tool for a certain disease. A tertiary prevention is an intervention that could prevent or reduce complications when a disease has declared itself. Tertiary preventions are important in the management of fatal diseases to improve the quality of life [5].

Imaging trials include a wide array of studies ranging from those used in screening of cancer or a disease, diagnosis in patients with symptoms or other clinical signs suggesting a problem, staging or evaluation of disease severity, evaluation of treatment, and detection of disease recurrence. Early trials may require a couple of dozen subjects to determine if an imaging modality appears to be useful, while more definitive phase III screening trials often require thousands of subjects and cost many millions of dollars.

Some clinical research focuses on the quality of life of patients. Those trials test new ways to decrease the severity of diseases or treatments. In the metastatic setting, the focus of clinical trials is to improve the quality of life and progression-free survival, which is different from studies with curative intent where the focus is to improve disease-free and overall survival. Chapter 11 discusses quality of life trials in detail.

2.3 Roles of different modalities

2.3.1 Surgery

Surgical removal remains the treatment of choice for the majority of solid tumors. Surgical oncologists play a very important role in both curative resections and palliation. A palliative procedure is performed in a patient who has metastatic disease, and the goal is to improve the quality of life for which palliation with pharmaceutical agents alone is not possible. The subject accepts the involved risks, and the general health of the subject allows for the intervention. Surgery to relieve bowel obstruction could fall into this category.

2.3.2 Radiation therapy

Compared with other treatment modalities like surgery and chemotherapy, radiation has the advantage of less toxicity. Radiation therapy aims at primary tumor for local disease, regional lymph nodes for locoregional disease, and systemic regions in metastasis.

In early-stage cancer, the higher dose of radiation is used with curative intent. With higher and more focused doses of radiation, considerable local control can be achieved [stereotactic radiation (SRT)].

In solid tumors where there is locoregional disease with lymph node involvement like lung cancer, radiation can target both the primary and locoregional lymph nodes with curative intent. Radiation with concurrent cisplatin-based chemotherapy can achieve higher efficacy and disease control.

In metastatic setting, palliative radiation can provide improvement in clinical symptoms. An example is palliative radiation to bony metastasis in breast and prostate cancer or whole brain radiation in cases of brain metastasis.

2.3.3 Chemotherapy combinations

Chemotherapy is the mainstay treatment of cancer. However, chemotherapy is associated with toxicity. A single agent or a combination of chemotherapeutic agents may be used. Chemotherapeutic agents can be used in combination with targeted therapy. They are used in curative, adjuvant, neoadjuvant, or palliative settings. In the curative setting, like treating non-Hodgkin lymphoma, the dose intensity is very important. In the adjuvant setting, such as treatment for breast, lung, or colorectal cancer after surgical resection, the benefit is determined by the risk of recurrence, which is based on patient demographics and tumor characteristics. In this setting, the adequate dosing is crucial [6].

In the neoadjuvant setting, the goal is to make the tumor resectable by giving systemic therapy before surgery, as is done for some breast, rectal, and pancreatic cancers. Furthermore, neoadjuvant treatment may improve outcome for some patients and tumor types compared to treatment after resection. If pathological complete response (pCR) occurs, the prognosis is good. A nice example is breast cancer where pCR indicates good prognosis and is being studied using early imaging assessment.

2.4 Study planning

2.4.1 Sources for protocol ideas

To generate a hypothesis, one needs to understand the biology, physiology, and epidemiology of the problem. In addition, one needs to consider the frustration due to unacceptable outcomes for patients [7]. The research idea or hypothesis can come from any activity within medicine. Some ideas are proposed by patho-physiology of a disease [5]. Some ideas about a new therapy or imaging approach have come from observations in clinic. Those observations could be shared with other people in the medical field through case reports, which could be just one case or a few cases [5]. For example, there was a case where a patient with Parkinson's disease taking amantadine to prevent influenza had remission for Parkinson's symptoms [8]. This case report led to a new treatment for Parkinson's. Other examples are tamoxifen, which was originally developed for contraception and is now used to prevent breast cancer, and azidothymidine (AZT), which originated as a potential agent to treat cancer and is now used to treat AIDS.

Many ideas come from trial and error. Population-based studies also provide ideas about prevention and treatments. For example, Burkitt observed that irritable bowel syndrome (IBS), colon cancer, and diverticulitis are less common in Africa than in developed countries that consume low-fiber diets. This observation led to the hypothesis about prevention of colon cancer with a high-fiber diet [5]. The main question or the hypothesis should not be answerable after all available literature has been reviewed. Feasibility of the question is another issue that needs to be considered, along with timing; premature research in humans can be risky and harm subjects. The transition from bench to bedside should not move too rapidly to avoid catastrophic adverse events [7].

The availability of a new device, such as a new scanner, or even a new analytic approach or software, regularly leads to comparisons with older methods. These often start as small phase II trials but can lead to very large phase III trials, such as the comparison of screen-film and digital mammography [9]. The application of a new imaging approach or therapy, which has been found to be efficacious in one disease or clinical situation, can often find utility in another disease.

The evaluation of new therapies may take advantage of novel imaging approaches, as described in Case example 1.2, Chapter 1. For example, metabolic imaging with ^{18}F-fluorodeoxyglucose or ^{18}F-3'-deoxy-3'-fluorothymidine-positron emission tomography (FDG PET or FLT PET) is being studied to assess response in multicenter trials. The goal is to determine if the change in uptake within 1–2 months predicts the ultimate treatment outcome and is now being compared to anatomic imaging or pCR in patients with breast cancer.

2.4.2 Choice of primary and secondary objectives

Before starting a research project, the primary objective needs to be clearly stated. Objectives should be specific and simple; after defining the primary objective, the secondary objectives should be stated. Sample size is calculated based on the primary objective [10] (see Section 7.5 for details on sample size calculation). The primary objective is the key; it will drive study design, statistic analysis, and accrual goals.

A surrogate endpoint, which could be a physical sign, a laboratory measurement, or an imaging finding, may be used as the study endpoint. A surrogate endpoint is easier, faster, and less expensive to study, while a long-term clinical endpoint, such as survival, might be difficult to measure. For example, measuring blood sugar could be a surrogate for complications or survival from diabetes; measuring cholesterol level could be a surrogate for atherosclerotic disease [11]. Clinical endpoints, such as pain, are sometimes difficult to measure since they are subjective; an X-ray of a joint can easily assess the inflammation or pain in a joint. However, the relationship between a clinically meaningful endpoint and a surrogate endpoint should be firmly established. A good example is pCR after neoadjuvant chemotherapy as a surrogate endpoint for breast cancer clinical trials, where the objective is to assess efficacy of new treatments to improve disease-free survival (DFS) (see Chapter 10 for definition of DFS). The relationship of pCR and prognosis and improved outcomes has been well established and has supported accelerated approval of new treatments for breast cancer by the FDA.

2.4.3 Ways to speed protocol writing

It is important to realize that a protocol is really an operational document and information for many sections can and should be copied from other sources. In general, the background section is the only part of the protocol that may be unique and should provide a succinct summary of the literature and rationale for a study. Some elements of the background may be obtained from grants written on the topic, but it must be kept in mind that grants are written to seek funding and are not meant to serve as a blueprint for the trial. Nonetheless, previous grants or manuscripts from the investigators may help in writing the background and rationale for a trial. The background section can also be helpful in writing future grants and the manuscript of the trials' results. The background information can be obtained in part by searching the usual web sites: *Pubmed* at http://www.ncbi.nlm.nih.gov/pubmed [12], *Radiological Society of North America (RSNA) journals* [13] at http://publications.rsna.org, and other sites. Knowledge and information about other similar trials can be obtained from national registries (http://clinicaltrials.gov/) [14]. It is important to know what other similar studies are being performed with similar patient populations, treatments, and imaging techniques.

When it comes to writing the many operational sections of a protocol, such as eligibility criteria, treatment and imaging schemes, and toxicity and risks, it is legitimate and useful to use similar trials as a template. One can often find full versions of trials from the above web sites, along with the National Cancer Institute (NCI), cooperative group sites (http://ctep.cancer.gov/ [15], http://www.acrin.org/ [16]), Google Web Search™, and with help from colleagues. Sometimes, the full protocols are posted with the understanding that other researchers should not have to "reinvent the wheel" when developing a trial. We often encourage investigators to replicate and revise standard descriptions of methods and side effects by using previous studies' protocols, publications, etc. Instruments for data collection also may be based on previous trials. For example, standard forms are available for quality of life, toxicity, and image interpretation. Consent forms also often contain a great deal of "boilerplate" text. Descriptions of methods, risks, benefits, HIPAA, and other sections are often standardized at a given institution, company, or cooperative group. In many cases, the consent form is actually put together by clinical trials office staff with oversight from the investigator. In general, consent forms are overly long, unreadable, and mostly unread by subjects [17]. Efforts have been underway to shrink consent from the usual 20–30 pages at present to a few succinct pages. To date, unfortunately, there has been little progress in this area.

2.4.4 Inclusion and exclusion criteria

The purpose of a clinical research study is to produce results that are applicable to other clinicians and institutions. To this end, the investigator designing a trial will want to include a group of subjects that will result in generalizable information; this requires careful thought in order to define the appropriate criteria to choose those to include in the study and those that should be eliminated from consideration. If the study group is defined too broadly, then one may find that the results will not be predictive for a specific patient; for example, a new staging test for patients with possible lung cancer detected on chest X-ray will have varying results and utility for patients with small solitary pulmonary nodules compared to those presenting with large masses and hilar adenopathy. Many patients in the first group may not even have cancer and those in the second will likely have advanced disease. If the patient population includes both groups, then the predictive value of a new test will greatly depend on the prior likelihood of each of the subsets of patients and the mix in the overall population. Such a broad group will not provide useful information for the clinician who may have a better sense of probability of a patient's stage based on the chest X-ray alone. Treatment studies face the same issues in determining if a new approach will be useful in a particular cancer, since the efficacy may greatly depend on histology, stage, molecular markers, and prior therapy. A new chemotherapy will have very different results, for example, in patients with advanced lung cancer, who have not received any prior chemotherapy, versus those who have failed all prior standard options [18]. Most studies of new drugs will clearly specify such criteria to include a more uniform group of identifiable patients.

On the other hand, if the study group is defined too narrowly, one may make inclusion criteria too specific, resulting in issues both in recruitment and generalizability. For example, if one eliminates subjects who have had significant diabetes from a trial in pancreatic cancer, one will eliminate many potential candidates, since the development of diabetes is often an early sign of the cancer [19]. Making such subjects ineligible will make recruitment more difficult and the results may not apply to such patients. Restrictions due to poor performance status are commonly included in therapeutic trials, since subjects with very poor function may stop a new drug early as they cannot tolerate any additional toxicity. On the other hand, if investigators only allow subjects who can walk up five flights of stairs, they will clearly do better, in part due to better tolerance of treatment, but they also have a lower disease burden. There is always a fine balance to maintain: one wants to eliminate subjects who are too sick or complex to tolerate the study and will not be evaluable for response and toxicity; on the other hand, one wants to include a broad enough group of subjects to make the results generally applicable.

2.4.4.1 Comorbid conditions

Subjects frequently have other prior conditions or ongoing clinical issues that need to be considered when assessing eligibility. Some of these need to be explicitly considered and described in the protocol. In some cases, we just assume that the clinician will not enroll a subject who clearly cannot participate or tolerate a protocol. For example, if an oral medication is included in a trial, subjects who cannot swallow pills may not be able to participate. This is generally not clearly stated, but assumed. In cancer trials, it is often stated that the subject cannot have any prior malignancy within the past 5 years, except for treated basal cell or squamous cell cancer of skin or treated *in situ* cervical cancer. Such requirements may be reasonable for adjuvant treatment trials but make little sense in subjects with advanced cancer where survival may be short. Medical problems in other organ systems are often explicitly described, for example, subjects with risk factors for heart disease are regularly excluded, including subjects with uncontrolled hypertension, unstable angina, recent myocardial infarction, or class III or IV heart failure. Often pulmonary or neurologic dysfunction is also precluded from enrollment.

2.4.4.2 Laboratory values

Screening laboratory values are regularly mandated for patients enrolling in clinical trials. These often include hematologic parameters (granulocytes, platelet count, hemoglobin) and renal function (creatinine) and liver function tests. It is very important to carefully think about every test that is ordered, since undoubtedly some subjects will have mild elevations of parameters, which may lead to exclusion. Depending on the test, one may allow for mild elevations. For example, the total bilirubin may be restricted to those less than or equal to 1.5 times the upper limit of normal, except in patients with Gilbert's syndrome. Depending on the laboratory, which often has the upper limit set at 1.5 mg/dl, this would mean that any value above 2.25 mg/dl would be excluded from the study. These limits may be different for subjects enrolled in studies who are known to have hepatitis or metastatic disease in the liver. It is important to exclude subjects where parameters clearly may affect safety. For example, subjects with renal dysfunction may be excluded since therapeutic drugs may be cleared more slowly leading to toxicity, while in imaging studies intravenous contrast may further impair renal function. In some imaging trials, investigators want to obtain renal and liver function tests, but the results do not determine eligibility. In such studies, the blood tests can be drawn prior to imaging, but the results do not need to be evaluated prior to enrollment in the study. Investigators must decide which tests are critical for safety and uniformity and which can be ignored. Since the general policy at this time is that *no waivers* are granted for tests out of range, one cannot simply ignore the results, but must exclude the subject. The timing of the tests must also be considered, since the results can change over time. Tests performed weeks in advance of the start of treatment may mean that important declines in organ function are missed. On the other hand, these tests must often be performed before registration, and for practical reasons, this generally needs to be done some days before the start of therapy. The compromise often leads to requiring baseline screening tests to be performed 7–14 days prior to the start of therapy.

2.4.4.3 Trial time requirements, risk, and accrual

Another issue in enrolling subjects on trials is the time and number of visits required to participate in a trial. Some subjects have constraints on their time, have transportation issues, or are generally unreliable in coming in for clinic visits. Even in the most responsible subjects, multiple visits may lead them to forgo enrollment on a clinical trial. Sometimes, exploration of novel imaging technologies will require additional time and slow the initiation of standard treatment, making patients less willing to participate. In part, the willingness of a subject to participate in such a trial will depend on their perceived benefits and risks. Multiple experimental imaging studies, which are added to the standard of care, but do not lead to known benefits, may impair enrollment. On the other hand, if investigators are enrolling subjects with refractory prostate cancer on a study of an experimental agent that has demonstrated exciting responses in an early trial, then enrollment may be very vigorous, despite the requirement of multiple research PET scans and tumor biopsies in addition to standard CT and bone scans.

2.4.5 Subject registration and accrual goals

The present regulations require that all consented subjects need to be accounted for and tracked. It is therefore important not to have subjects sign consent until eligibility for full protocol participation is considered likely. Most standard of care evaluations that can be completed without consent should be obtained prior to signing consent. While one may discuss the protocol, present the consent form, and go over the procedures, risks, and benefits, it is best not to have the subject sign consent prior to considering eligibility and assessing the subject's desire to fully participate in the study. Depending on the wording in the protocol, one may even need to file adverse event reports for consented subjects who have not undergone any study-specific procedures or treatments. Many studies include evaluations that are not standard of care prior to determining eligibility to participate in treatment. In such cases, it is essential that the consent form is signed before such tests are performed.

There is often a difference between the number of subjects consented and the final number of evaluable patients. The Institutional Review Board (IRB) often base the accrual target on the number of consented subjects, so it is important to take into account the likely number of subjects who may be screen failures, or not complete enough of the study to be evaluable. Many therapeutic studies are based on the intention to treat, which can mean that once a subject is randomized to one arm of a treatment trial, they will be followed for response. On the other

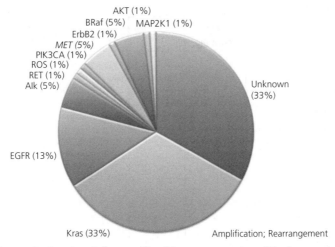

AKT (1%)
BRaf (5%) MAP2K1 (1%)
ErbB2 (1%)
MET (5%)
PIK3CA (1%)
ROS (1%)
RET (1%)
Alk (5%)

Unknown
(33%)

EGFR (13%)

Kras (33%)   Amplification; Rearrangement

Figure 2.2 Genetic alterations in non-small-cell lung cancer and possible therapeutic targets. Source: Gerold Bepler. Reproduced with permission from Gerold Bepler. Data sources: FDA [21] and Gallin [22]. © Gerold Bepler.

hand, if one is doing a study looking at a change in two images over time, then clearly those who miss the second imaging session are not evaluable, but still must be counted as study participants. Planning for accrual goals must take such situations into account, and the target number of subjects for a study should generally take into consideration dropouts. In some therapeutic studies using targeted agents, a particular genetic characteristic is required for patients who are going to receive treatment. For example, in subjects with lung cancer, the ALK gene rearrangement is present in about 5% of subjects, so studies demonstrating the efficacy of crizotinib can require screening hundreds of subjects [20] (Figure 2.2). A separate consent form just for the genetic screening test is often employed, while subjects who are positive then have another treatment consent form to sign. These distinct groups of subjects must be described in the protocol and taken into account in the accrual goals.

2.4.6 Evaluation schedule

Trial complexity has increased enormously over the last couple of decades. This is evident both in the eligibility criteria, as noted earlier, and also in the evaluation tests performed pretreatment and during the protocol. More frequent tumor biopsies are needed, including recent biopsies of metastatic lesions to ensure that heterogeneity in the tumor or changes over time have not altered the genomics of the cancer and hence the choice of treatment. During therapy repeated biopsies are more commonly performed in early-stage trials to ensure that the target has been modulated by the therapy. Sophisticated imaging tests are also included in many studies (PET, SPECT, MRI) to measure physiologic tumor parameters and changes with treatment. The toxicities of the specific therapeutic agents have also

Study calendar

Cycle	1	2			3		4
Prestudy	13*	21	34*	39*	42	55*	63
Treatment							
Liposomal doxorubicin		X	X			X		X
Physical							
History and physical exam	X		X			X		X
Weight and performance status	X		X					X
Tumor measurement (CT/MR)	X				X			
Toxicity notation	X		X			X		X
Laboratory							
CBC with differential, platelets	X	X	X	X		X	X	X
Multiphasic	X		X			X		X
CEA (every other cycle)	X					X		

*± 3 days.

Figure 2.3 Sample study schedule from a simple phase II trial of liposomal doxorubicin in refractory colon cancer [23]. Source: Data from Ethgen [23].

led to baseline and repeated evaluation of normal organs, for example, ophthalmologic exams, pulmonary function tests, ECGs, and cardiac evaluation. This is beyond all the routine blood counts and chemistry tests that are performed, along with an expanding list of other blood tests and pharmacologic monitoring.

2.4.7 Treatment schedule

During the course of the trial, the schedule for treatment and evaluation must be carefully laid out (Figure 2.3). It is important to describe the optimal treatment schedule but also consider and allow alterations in the schedule when needed. Clearly, toxicity or medical complications may require changes in the treatment schedule (Section 2.4.9). One must also account for issues such as holidays, subject's vacation, and inclement weather. Allowing some minor variation (e.g., ±2 days) in the exact treatment schedule is helpful and will minimize struggles that occur every year between Thanksgiving and the New Year. Blood tests and scans must also be carefully timed. For example, requiring that a follow-up scan be performed on day 55, rather than during the week prior to treatment, may lead to scheduling problems and unnecessary deviations.

2.4.8 Assessment of toxicity and reporting adverse events

Assessment of safety as well as efficacy is important in clinical research. It is easy to evaluate the safety and occurrence of well-known adverse events, like neutropenia due to chemotherapy, which is a well-known side effect. However, it is more difficult to evaluate unusual or rare adverse events of a new medication or procedure.

According to the FDA, an adverse event is any undesirable experience that is associated with the use of a medicine or procedure in a subject. Serious adverse events must be reported to the FDA if the outcome is one of the following: death, a life-threatening event, hospitalization, disability or permanent damage, birth defect requiring intervention to prevent permanent impairment or damage, or other serious important medical events [24]. Serious adverse events must also be reported to the sponsor and IRB; the reporting time should be stated in the protocol [25].

All adverse events in the clinical trials should be documented even if the event appears not to be related to the clinical research intervention [25]. The Common Terminology Criteria for Adverse Events (CTCAE) version 4.0 that was developed by the NCI is a good guideline for adverse events. The NCI's guideline describes the adverse events and categorizes them by severity (grade) and organ. All versions of CTCAE are available from this web site (http://ctep.cancer.gov/ protocolDevelopment/electronic_applications/ctc.htm#ctc_40) and applications for smart phones or tablets are also available.

There can also be unexpected events that are not listed in the consent form, the protocol, or in the brochure [25]. Since the occurrence of unexpected events is more common than the term implies, investigators need to find methods to recognize unexpected events and their association with treatment, for example, benoxaprofen-induced hepatorenal disease or thalidomide-induced phocomelia.

There were 548 new chemicals that were approved by the FDA between 1970 and 2000. About 10.2% of those new agents caused serious adverse events, about 2.9% were withdrawn from the market, and in 8.2% warnings needed to be added to their labeling. Overall, randomized clinical trials perform poorly in detecting adverse events [3]. Evidence across different medical fields suggests that reporting harm data in trials is inadequate [26]. One of the reasons for poorly identified and reported harm data is that a trial does not commence with a goal to show that a new intervention has more adverse events; usually the focus is on the positive events, and time and effort are spent to demonstrate that. In addition, rare and serious adverse events will be detected only after a large number of subjects are exposed to the medication or procedure. During a phase III trial, typically with fewer subjects than a phase IV trial, rare adverse effects have very low probability of being detected. However, there is a higher chance of detecting rare adverse events in a postmarketing surveillance [3].

Underreporting harm data can cause unnecessary morbidities and mortalities. Incomplete evidence can lead to incorrect conclusions about new interventions; therefore, underreporting harm data can result in overestimating the benefits and underestimating the risks of new treatments [27]. Overall, underreporting clinical trial findings is unethical and unscientific [28].

2.4.9 Scheme for dose modification

A clinical trial of a therapy must specify the basic dose schedule, route of administration, amount and frequency of dosage, and also which nonprotocol drugs are permissible and under what circumstances. Before the conduct of a phase I trial, investigators sometimes conduct exploratory microdosing phase 0 studies. These involve very limited subjects and should be performed in 7 days or less at 1/50th to 1/100th the dose that showed no adverse effects in preclinical toxicology studies. These studies allow for the assessment of drug clearance and comparison to those performed in animals and help set the starting dose for phase I trials. The phase I study goal is to obtain the maximum tolerated dose (MTD) and to determine an appropriate dose for the next phase in study. Phase I starts with a very low dose and increases in preplanned steps. The maximum recommended starting dose for new agents is generally calculated by determining the *human equivalent dose (HED)* for the *no observed adverse effect levels (NOAELs)* in an animal and then dividing by a safety factor of 10 or greater [29].

One common scheme is that if there is no *dose limiting toxicity (DLT)* in a cohort of three to six subjects, the dose is escalated for the next cohort. DLT is the dose that side effects appear during treatment. If DLT is seen in 33% of subjects, then three more subjects are treated at the same dose level. If no more DLT is seen, then the dose will be escalated for the next cohort. If the DLT is more than 33% at a dose level, the dose escalation stops.

The phase II trial usually is set as the highest dose for which the incidence of DLT is less than 33% [30]. Dose modification frequently occurs in clinical trials. Dose reduction is the most common type of dose modification; however, increased doses have been used as well. For example, in the clinical trial of chronic myelogenous leukemia, which used imatinib in the intervention arm, imatinib's initial dose was 400 mg/day; however, some subjects did not show significant response in 3 months. The dose was then increased to 400 mg twice daily in subjects without adverse events [31]. Dose reductions are allowed in some phase III clinical trials; for example, in a phase III clinical trial comparing single agent docetaxel with capecitabine and docetaxel in advanced breast cancer [32], the dose modification was used extensively in the combination arm.

Dose reduction or delays usually happen following an intolerable adverse event. It is important to provide instructions in the study protocol for dose reduction and delays, or removing the subject from the study in case an adverse event occurs. A dose reduction scheme in the study protocol allows the investigator to reduce the dose, if needed. Without any sufficient instruction in the protocol, either the study subject needs to be discontinued or the protocol needs a time-consuming amendment [33]. When unexpected need arises due to safety issues, it is permissible to alter or stop treatment and inform the IRB and FDA while the protocol is being amended and approved.

2.4.10 Data collection and documentation

The data collected during a clinical trial needs to be accurate and the database needs to be secure. Before data collection begins, all clinical trials should have a *data management plan (DMP)*, which provides guidance for handling data in all circumstances. DMP is a document that should be developed before data collection and should define all activities related to data collection from the beginning until database closeout. The DMP should comply with all regulatory guidelines and laws. The goal for data collection is to provide a database for the study, which is secure, reliable, accurate, and ready for analysis. A meaningful analysis requires collecting the correct data points. Missing data, incorrect data, and excess variability need to be avoided.

The *case report form (CRF)* is a document for capturing data in clinical trials. CRFs used to be paper based. While electronic data capture (EDC) has increased, paper-based forms are still used when EDC is impossible for financial reasons [34].

The details of subject information that need to be recorded should be stated in the study protocol. CRFs provide data that will eventually be analyzed and lead to the clinical trial results. Therefore, accuracy of data collection depends on appropriate forms. Information that is not included in the form will not be available at the end of study. In addition, the collection of too much data from each subject can be challenging and costly [2]. Questions in the form should be easy to understand. Double negative and compound questions should be avoided and precise questions need to be asked. Forms should be unambiguous and quick to complete. In Case example 1.2 (Chapter 1), where evaluation of treatment response is being studied, one needs to carefully document the amount of therapy actually received and its timing. Furthermore, the patient outcome also needs to be included with dates, standard clinical imaging evaluation, and measurements by RECIST 1.1, in addition to corresponding PET assessments. Development of the data form is a collaborative effort that usually requires months of work. One common problem is that investigators want to create forms to meet the clinical research goal and also for routine patient care. Investigators should realize that the information for day-to-day patient care is not necessary for research and the data about primary and secondary outcomes of the clinical trial must be in the form [35]. In a clinical trial, it is usually imperative to enroll subjects as fast as possible. Therefore, a fundamental concept in a clinical trial is to keep the data collection form as brief as possible; for example, in the ISIS-1 study of intravenous atenolol among 16,027 cases of suspected acute myocardial infarction, the investigators collected only enough data to fill a single page for each case. This approach allowed the enrollment of many subjects with no reimbursement to health providers enrolling subjects. This trial discovered a very important finding in cardiovascular disease [25].

Finally, the data should be kept in a locked and protected location with adequate backup [35].

2.5 The protocol review process

All subject research protocols require a regulatory review that often takes months to accomplish. The present goal at many institutions is to move protocols for submission to activation in under 3 months, but this can be difficult for many

Table 2.1 Protocol submission documents.

Protocol
Consent Form
HIPAA Authorization Form
Protocol Submission Form for Scientific Review and Approval Form
Protocol Submission Form for Institutional Review Board
Radiation Safety Form
Drug Use Form
Package Inserts for Drugs
Investigational Drug Brochures
Biologic Specimen Form
Documentation of Personnel on the Protocol including CVs, conflict of interest, and research training documentation
Any Forms, instructions, surveys, or logs given to participants
Advertisements or recruiting materials for physicians and patients
Forms for special populations: children, pregnant women, prisoners, and those with diminished capacity

reasons, and it is often not under the control of the investigator or even the research institution. The list of documents and forms needed for submission for review can be daunting (Table 2.1). The first step is often a protocol review committee in the department or research center that judges the protocol for scientific and clinical validity, feasibility in terms of resources available and funding, competing protocols, and the ability to recruit the needed number of subjects. A statistical review should also be conducted at this point. Once the protocol is completed by the research team, it will be submitted for review to the IRB, which works to oversee the safety, rights, and well-being of research subjects. The IRB will include clinicians, scientists, and laypeople. They will review the consent form in detail to assure that the research subject is well informed of the procedures, risks, and benefits of the study.

It is rare that a protocol does not require revision during its execution. Amendments are often submitted when inconsistent operational descriptions are encountered once the study is underway and alterations are needed to simplify the protocol. Adverse events may lead to a change in treatment as well as altering the informed consent to describe the problem to the subjects.

Once protocols are open, they generally undergo annual IRB review to assess progress. They are often audited to ensure that eligibility criteria are being met and study procedures are being followed. All appropriate documentation is critical to this process. The clinical chart and records must tell a complete story of the subject's participation in the study. If it is not recorded on paper or in a secured computer source, there is no proof that the study was properly conducted. (See Chapter 6 for more details about operational aspects of conducting a clinical trial.)

2.6 Funding and budgeting

Clinical research is expensive and has become more so with the increased complexity of clinical trials. For example, a phase II study in refractory colorectal patients conducted a decade ago using liposomal doxorubicin cost about $3000 per subject. Such trials are rarely performed nowadays. A recent study of similar subjects as part of an expansion cohort in a phase I study budgeted about $30,000 per subject. Funding sources play a critical role in research. These can include internal seed money grants to get preliminary data, while larger studies will require funding from the NIH or pharmaceutical manufacturers. The NIH offers very competitive funding through large grants to individual investigators or multi-investigator programs. Grants are also offered in conjunction with small businesses. When budgeting for such trials, it is important to take into account the many costs involved in a study. This includes start-up costs, such as the investigators' time, regulatory, and review costs. Physician and nurse time in recruiting and following subjects along with costs of data collection and management must be included. Laboratory or imaging studies that are not part of the standard of care need to be included in the budget.

2.7 Enhancing protocol accrual

Recruitment is the most significant rate-limiting step in a clinical trial. The golden rule is that about half of the planned sample size will be recruited in twice the time that was anticipated.

Many patients who are eligible for a clinical trial refuse to participate. There are several reasons for low recruitment in clinical trials. Some of them are lack of awareness, enrollment obstacles, barriers to ethnic minorities and economically disadvantaged, elderly barriers, and physician-related barriers.

Lack of awareness is one of the main barriers in recruiting subjects to the study. About 40% of adults do not have any idea about clinical research and how clinical trials are performed. Based on a survey conducted by the NCI, 85% of patients who had a malignancy were not aware of clinical trials, but 75% of them were willing to participate if they had information about them. Patients don't know that participating in clinical trials is free. Patients don't have any knowledge about clinical trials, so they don't ask about them.

Fear of the study is one of the enrollment barriers for patients. Patients refuse to enroll in studies because there is fear and mistrust toward investigators. Patients are also concerned about the cost of the study and harm they might incur. Another enrollment obstacle is rigid protocols with strict eligibility criteria. Therefore, many patients are disqualified for that reason. Lack of time, childcare, and transportation also prevent patients from enrolling in clinical trials.

Minorities are underrepresented in clinical trials. There is fear and mistrust in medical research among minorities. In addition, there are fewer minority healthcare providers to recruit minority subjects. Medically underserved and economically disadvantaged people have similar difficulties. For example, patients without insurance participate less in clinical trials, while patients with higher socioeconomic level have higher clinical trial accrual rates.

Physicians refer elderly patients less often to clinical trials. History of prior cancer, comorbid conditions, lack of transportation, and difficulty with compliance are other obstacles for recruiting the elderly. The majority of protocols exclude elderly from participation.

Many physicians never refer patients to clinical trials. Many doctors are unfamiliar and unaware of clinical trials. Some protocols are so rigid that physicians don't refer patients. Some physicians cannot justify the risk and benefit of new interventions. Lack of time and resources are other reasons not to offer trials to patients [36, 37].

There are a number of strategies to improve trial recruitment. These include performing a feasibility study before the larger trial, keeping the study eligibility broad, avoiding competition between studies, adding more recruiting sites, advertising the trial directly to potential subjects through posters, and optimizing the clinical trial experience for both subjects and researchers.

Public knowledge about clinical trials needs to improve. Healthcare providers need to provide clear information without any technical and complex terminology. The cost of participating in clinical trials should be communicated to potential subjects. Families of patients should be involved and educated in clinical trials; social workers should also be involved. More information needs to be provided to physicians about ongoing clinical trials, and a research network of physicians needs to be developed. Use of technology and the Internet can promote and improve recruitment of subjects to clinical trials.

References

1 Kummar, S., et al., Phase 0 clinical trials: conceptions and misconceptions. *Cancer J,* 2008. **14**(3): p. 133–137.
2 Pocock, S.J., *Clinical Trials, 1st ed.* 1983, John Wiley & Sons: Chichester.
3 Haynes, R.B., et al., *Clinical Epidemiology: How To Do Clinical Practice Research, 3rd ed.* 2006, Lippincott Williams & Wilkins: Philadelphia, PA.
4 Zia, M., et al., Comparison of outcomes of phase II studies and subsequent randomized control studies using identical chemotherapeutic regimens. *J Clin Oncol,* 2005. **23**(28): p. 6982–6991.
5 Fletcher, R. and S. Fletcher, *Clinical Epidemiology, 4th ed.* 2005, Lippincott Williams & Wilkins: Baltimore, MA.
6 Schrijvers, D., et al., *Handbook of Cancer in the Senior Patients, 1st ed.* 2010, ESMO: New York.
7 Derenzo, E. and J. Moss, *Writing Clinical Research Protocol, 1st ed.* 2006, Elsevier Academic Press: Burlington, MA.

8 Schwab, R.S., et al., Amantadine in the treatment of Parkinson's disease. *JAMA*, 1969. **208**(7): p. 1168–1170.

9 Pisano, E., et al., Diagnostic performance of digital versus film mammography for breast-cancer screening. *N Engl J Med*, 2005. **353**(17): p. 1773–1783.

10 PennState Eberly College of Science, Design and Analysis of Clinical Trials 2014. 2014; Available from: https://onlinecourses.science.psu.edu/stat509/node/31 (accessed September 2, 2015).

11 Sullivan, E. Clinical Trial Endpoint. FDA, Editor. 2014; Available from: http://www.fda.gov/downloads/Training/ClinicalInvestigatorTrainingCourse/UCM283378.pdf (accessed August 15, 2015).

12 U.S. National Library of Medicine National Institutes of Health, 2014; Available from: http://www.ncbi.nlm.nih.gov/pubmed (accessed March 20, 2014).

13 RadioGraphics, R., 2014; Available from: http://pubs.rsna.org (accessed March 20, 2014).

14 Clinical Trials.gov A service fo the U.S. National Institutes of Health, 2014; Available from: http://clinicaltrials.gov (accessed March 20, 2014).

15 National Cancer Institute CTEP (Cancer Therapy Evaluation Program), 2014; Available from: http://ctep.cancer.gov (accessed March 20, 2014).

16 American College of Radiology Imaging Network (ACRIN), 2014; Available from: http://www.acrin.org (accessed March 20, 2014).

17 Desch, K., et al., Analysis of informed consent document utilization in a minimal-risk genetic study. *Ann Intern Med*, 2011. **155**(5): p. 316–322.

18 Shaw, A.T., et al., Crizotinib versus chemotherapy in advanced ALK-positive lung cancer. *N Engl J Med*, 2013. **368**(25): p. 2385–2394.

19 Wang, F., S. Gupta, and E.A. Holly, Diabetes mellitus and pancreatic cancer in a population-based case-control study in the San Francisco Bay Area, California. *Cancer Epidemiol Biomarkers Prev*, 2006. **15**(8): p. 1458–1463.

20 Soda, M., et al., Identification of the transforming EML4-ALK fusion gene in non-small-cell lung cancer. *Nature*, 2007. **448**(7153): p. 561–566.

21 FDA, What is a Serious Adverse Event. 2004; Available from: http://www.fda.gov/safety/medwatch/howtoreport/ucm053087.htm (accessed August 15, 2015).

22 Gallin, J. and F. Ognibene, *Principles and Practice of Clinical Research, 2nd ed.* 2007, Elsevier Academic Press: Burlington, MA.

23 Ethgen, M., et al., Reporting of harm in randomized, controlled trials of nonpharmacologic treatment for rheumatic disease. *Ann Intern Med*, 2005. **143**(1): p. 20–25.

24 Mahinbakht, A., S.M. Lavasani, and M. Guirguis, The quality of reporting harms-related data in clinical trials of adjuvant trastuzumab in early-stage breast cancer treatment. *Ther Innov Regul Sci*, 2014. **48**(3): p. 299–304.

25 Dickersin, K. and I. Chalmers. Recognising, Investigating and Dealing with Incomplete and Biased Reporting of Clinical Research: From Francis Bacon to the World Health Organisation. JLL Bulletin: Commentaries on the History of Treatment Evaluation. 2010; Available from: http://www.jameslindlibrary.org/illustrating/articles/recognising-investigating-and-dealing-with-incomplete-and-biase (accessed August 15, 2015).

26 FDA, Guidance for Industry Estimating the Maximum Safe Starting Dose in Initial Clinical Trials for Therapeutics in Adult Healthy Volunteers. 2005. http://www.fda.gov/downloads/Drugs/Guidances/UCM078932.pdf (accessed September 16, 2015).

27 DeVita, V., T. Lawrence, and S. Rosenbert, *Cancer Principles & Practice of Oncology, 8th ed.* 2008, Lippincott William & Wilkins: Philadelphia, PA.

28 O'Brien, S.G., et al., Imatinib compared with interferon and low-dose cytarabine for newly diagnosed chronic-phase chronic myeloid leukemia. *N Engl J Med*, 2003. **348**(11): p. 994–1004.

29 O'Shaughnessy, J., et al., Superior survival with capecitabine plus docetaxel combination therapy in anthracycline-pretreated patients with advanced breast cancer: phase III trial results. *J Clin Oncol*, 2002. **20**(12): p. 2812–2823.

30 Brody, T., *Clinical Trials Study Design, Endpoints and Biomarkers, Drug Safety and FDA and ICH Guidelines, 1st ed.* 2012, Elsevier Inc.: London.

31 Richesson, R.L. and P. Nadkarni, Data standards for clinical research data collection forms: current status and challenges. *J Am Med Inform Assoc*, 2011. **18**(3): p. 341–346.

32 Weinstein, J.N. and R.A. Deyo, Clinical research: issues in data collection. *Spine (Phila Pa 1976)*, 2000. **25**(24): p. 3104–3109.

33 The Cochrane Collaboration, Cochrane Handbook for Systematic Reviews of Interventions Version 5.1.0. 2011; Available from: www.cochrane-handbook.org (accessed August 15, 2015).

34 Williams, S., *Clinical Trials Recruitment and Enrollment: Attitudes, Barriers, and Motivating Factors*. A Summary of Literature and Market Research Reports Held by NCI. August 2004. Retrieved from http://cro.rbhs.rutgers.edu/documents/clinical_trials_recruitment_and_enrollment.pdf (accessed September 16, 2015).

35 Li, T., et al., Genotyping and genomic profiling of non-small-cell lung cancer: implications for current and future therapies. *J Clin Oncol*, 2013. **31**(8): p. 1039–1049.

36 Pao, W. and N. Girard, New driver mutations in non-small-cell lung cancer. *Lancet Oncol*, 2011. **12**(2): p. 175–180.

37 Shields, A., L. Lange, and M. Zalupski, Phase II study of liposomal doxorubicin in patients with advanced colorectal cancer. *Am J Clin Oncol*, 2001. **24**(1): p. 96–98.

CHAPTER 3

Clinical trials of image-guided interventions including radiotherapy studies

Gary S. Dorfman[1] and Stephen M. Hahn[2]

[1] Weill Cornell Medical College, New York, NY, USA
[2] The University of Texas MD Anderson Cancer Center, Houston, TX, USA

KEY POINTS

- Clinical trials of local–regional, image-guided, device-mediated interventions have associated characteristics, caveats, and pitfalls, some of which are similar to and others that are different from clinical trials of drug and biological agents.

- The evidence required for FDA clearance and/or approval of medical devices may be different from and insufficient to support specific clinical utilities. Therefore, clinical trials of local–regional device-mediated interventions and the associated imaging guidance are necessary to achieve widespread availability of such interventions in clinical care.

- The design and conduct of clinical trials of image-guided, local–regional, device-mediated interventions demand an understanding of concepts specific to the stage of translation of the intervention, the disease, and the intended clinical utility of the intervention as well as the device or devices employed in the intervention.

- Clinical trials of image-guided, local–regional, device-mediated interventions must include mechanisms to measure and control for the differences among devices and for the role of the operator(s).

3.1 Introduction

This chapter will discuss important aspects of clinical trials of image-guided interventions (IGI), herein defined as *in vivo*, minimally or noninvasive, device-based diagnostic and therapeutic procedures that utilize real-time imaging for targeting, monitoring, and assessment of intraprocedural endpoint determination. In addition, the imaging modalities used (e.g., MRI, CT, ultrasound (US), PET, NM, fluoroscopy, optical, and combinations of these) provide information beyond what is visible by natural light and the operator's vision (whether unaided or aided by

---

Handbook for Clinical Trials of Imaging and Image-Guided Interventions, First Edition.
Edited by Nancy A. Obuchowski and G. Scott Gazelle.
© 2016 John Wiley & Sons, Inc. Published 2016 by John Wiley & Sons, Inc.

various types of "scopes" such as operative microscopes, angioscopes, or endoscopes). The overwhelming majority of IGI are local or regional, rather than systemic, procedures. The interventions may be open, percutaneous, transvascular, endoluminal, or noninvasive, external application of energy (e.g., radiation therapy or focused US). These local or regional interventions also may activate or may be potentiated by systemically administered pharmacologic, biologic, or immunologic agents. We do not include within the definition of IGI local or regional device-based procedures that use imaging solely for subject selection, planning the intervention, or assessment of response at times temporally separate from the intervention itself. Of course, IGI and trials of such interventions certainly may include imaging for selection of subjects, procedural planning, and/or response assessment in addition to the use of real-time imaging for targeting, procedural monitoring, and intraprocedural endpoint determination.

While the chapter provides information about IGI trials, some of which are in common with other types of clinical trials, greatest attention is devoted to the specifics of such trials that differentiate them from trials of systemic pharmacologic and biologic agents, local or regional therapies that do not use real-time imaging (e.g., most open surgeries or endoscopic procedures), and trials of imaging for purposes outside of real-time imaging during the procedure (such as screening, diagnosis, or response assessment).

An important point to consider at the outset is why trials of IGI are even important in an era that is becoming defined by "personalized medicine" based on systemically administered "targeted pharmacologic and biologic" therapies. First, while there are some targeted therapies available, many more are required to address the plethora of targets important in various specific disease states. It takes many years and significant financial investment to translate targeted therapies from conception to clinical delivery. Second, even when targeted therapies are available, it is difficult to completely control diffuse disease without the inclusion of neoadjuvant and/or adjuvant, local and regional therapies for use in specific anatomic sites. For example, most nonhematologic malignancies require local or regional intervention in addition to systemic treatment. The same is true for many instances of atherosclerotic vascular diseases, degenerative diseases, and congenital diseases. Third, even systemically administered targeted therapies may have undesirable nontarget adverse effects. When locally restricted predisease or early disease is discovered (perhaps by screening programs), it may be more effective and less intrusive to eradicate such local pathology with a minimally or noninvasive local intervention, such as an IGI. This paradigm is already embraced for the prevention of squamous cell carcinoma by the local eradication of actinic keratoses. One could easily imagine the extension of this paradigm to anatomies not so easily accessible by the use of various advanced imaging modalities and available or yet to be developed local/regional IGI and to nononcologic diseases.

Currently many available local and regional device-based therapies are performed using open surgical, endoscopic, or radiation therapy techniques that do not use real-time imaging guidance. Therefore, there may be an opportunity to improve patient outcomes by improving the effectiveness and reducing the intrusiveness of local and regional therapies through the uses of real-time imaging inherent in IGIs. For such IGIs to be available to patients, it is important that compelling evidence defining the appropriate use of the IGI in specific clinical conditions is made available. The development of such evidence is dependent on appropriately designed and properly conducted clinical trials, recognizing the unique aspects inherent in clinical trials of IGIs.

3.2 Establishing the context for IGI clinical trials

3.2.1 Clinical utilities

IGI may be targeted toward a variety of clinical purposes or utilities. Using oncologic interventions as an example, potential clinical utilities might include the following:

1 **Secondary palliation** in which the targeted intervention provides palliation of symptoms without directly attacking the underlying tumor burden (e.g., percutaneous nephrostomy, gastrostomy, biliary drainage)
2 **Primary palliation** in which the intent is palliation by directly targeting specific sites of tumor causing the underlying symptom of clinical concern (e.g., ablation of bony metastases by irradiation therapy or ablative techniques such as radiofrequency, microwave, or cryotherapy; embolotherapy of symptomatic hepatic neuroendocrine tumors)
3 **Adjunctive interventions** to supplement or potentiate local or systemic therapies (e.g., preoperative portal vein embolization, venous access to allow delivery of systemic pharmacotherapy, embolotherapy of hepatic metastases from colorectal carcinoma with curative intent or to improve time to progression-/disease-free survival duration)
4 **Neoadjuvant interventions** as a component of a treatment plan with curative intent (e.g., ablative intervention of focal hepatocellular carcinoma as a bridge to transplantation)
5 **Primary curative interventions** generally for localized early-stage disease or for eradicating predisease (e.g., in circumstances where the cost-effectiveness of IGI eradication of predisease or early disease is favorable in comparison with continued monitoring of the sentinel lesion including diagnostic work-up culminating in eventual treatment)

Aspects of an IGI toward which a clinical trial might be targeted include one or more of the following:

1 Performance of the inherent imaging modalities used for real-time targeting, monitoring, and intraprocedural endpoint determination
2 Visualization/localization enhancers (e.g., contrast agents, mechanisms sensitive to pH or temperature)
3 Computational methods to improve targeting and tracking (e.g., motion and respiratory compensation)

4 Methods of improving real-time image and signal processing

5 Navigation and procedural control tools such as robotics

6 Effectors of the actual intervention (e.g., ablation probes, embolic agents, catheters, biopsy instruments, stents)

7 Integration of various tools and techniques as enumerated above

8 Comparison between the performance of different treatment paradigms for a given clinical condition and for one of the previously enumerated clinical utilities (e.g., relative performance of two different IGIs, relative performance of an IGI with or without an additional systemic intervention, relative performance of a systemic intervention with or without a concomitant IGI, relative performance of an IGI as compared with some other standard of care treatment)

3.2.2 Translational continuum

There is a generally agreed upon translational continuum leading from basic discovery or an applied engineering concept to the availability of an effective clinical intervention. The stages of this continuum relative to an IGI are outlined in Table 3.1. This continuum describes the "vertical" translation from an initial discovery or concept to clinical utility and availability. In addition, a not infrequent scenario is the "horizontal" translation of an existing IGI from one clinical utility to another. Such a translation might still benefit from a rigorous data-driven continuum involving some or all of the steps in Table 3.1.

Additionally, clinical trials evaluating the use of imaging in subject (patient) selection, treatment planning, and postprocedural monitoring for response assessment and evaluation of potential adverse events may be of interest. These additional foci of investigation are similar to the evaluation of imaging for these same utilities in the context of systemic therapies and traditional local/regional therapies that do not employ real-time image guidance. However, as will be discussed subsequently in this chapter, one must recognize that there are important differences to such evaluations in the context of IGIs.

The design of an IGI trial will be influenced by (i) the intended clinical utility(ies) toward which the IGI will be applied, (ii) the specific aspect(s) of the IGI chosen for investigation, (iii) the stage of maturity of the IGI along the

Table 3.1 Stages of translational continuum for an IGI.

1 Basic science discovery or applied engineering concept

2 Optimization

3 Feasibility/safety/local biologic effect

4 Validation for specific applications

5 Regulatory approval

6 Supportive payer policies promulgated

7 Widespread physician acceptance

8 Patient recognition and "informed" demand (with unsafe or ineffective interventions withdrawn and/or reworked through the preceding steps of the translational continuum)

translational continuum, and (iv) most obviously the disease(s) or clinical condition(s) within which the IGI will used. Thus, the design and conduct of clinical trials to study IGIs have much in common with trials of interventions generally and surgical interventions more specifically (since surgical interventions are a widely recognized subset of local/regional interventions) and also commonalities with trials of imaging modalities (see Chapter 1), but there are critical differences. This chapter will explore the important areas of commonality and stress those areas of critical differences between IGI trials and other therapy trials as well as between IGI trials and other types of imaging trials.

3.2.3 Why do IGI clinical trials differ from other therapy or imaging trials?

As discussed in Chapter 2, clinical trials of systemically administered interventions (pharmacologic or biologic) are organized into well-defined phases (Phase 0–IV) defined by the FDA, with trial design in each of the phases largely based on the maturity of the intervention for the intended clinical purpose and the intended objectives of the trial. Since devices are regulated very differently from drugs and biologics, including oversight by a different center (Center for Devices and Radiological Health (CDRH)) within the FDA, the paradigm presented in Chapter 2 does not apply to device trials including, but not limited to, trials of IGI devices. Device trials, when demanded for regulatory approval, are defined by a paradigm with two broad classes, Pilot and Pivotal. In actual practice it is a very small minority of devices that include clinical trials for specific clinical indications as part of the regulatory pathway to commercialization. Devices are classified by the FDA into one of three classes (http://www.fda.gov/MedicalDevices/DeviceRegulationandGuidance/ Overview/ClassifyYourDevice/default.htm), and the majority of devices employed for IGIs fall within Class 2. Nearly all of the devices in Class 2 are not approved by the FDA but instead are cleared through a Premarket Notification process, commonly known as the 510(k) pathway, based on demonstration of substantial equivalency to a previously cleared device or device(s). This demonstration of substantial equivalency may or may not involve clinical trials, and should such trials be included among the evidence provided to the FDA, their design is usually quite different from trials of pharmacologic or biologic interventions; and necessarily so as the stated primary and secondary objectives/endpoints are usually quite different.

Even trials designed to support the approval (not clearance as is the case for Class 2 devices) of Class 3 devices (so called Pivotal trials) have substantial design differences. Some have questioned the rigor of such device approval trials [1]. Others have justified the majority of the trial design differences as necessary and inherent in the differences between drugs/biologics and devices as outlined to follow. The Institute of Medicine, in a recent review of the 510(k) mechanism, remained silent on the issue of Class 3 device evaluation utilizing the Premarket Approval (PMA) process [2]. But the report does acknowledge the important differences in general between the drug/biologic and the device ecosystems. Not widely or definitively addressed to date is the effect that the lack of a rigorous, progressive, and granular clinical trial hierarchy (e.g., such as Phase 0–IV as is used for trials of drugs and biologics) has on trials of medical devices. A detailed analysis of the device regulatory pathways is beyond the scope of this text, but an in-depth understanding of this topic is recommended for the trialist interested in pursuing IGI clinical trials.

However, the current healthcare delivery system demands data on which evidence-based decision-making is based. In the case of pharmacologic and bio-logic (systemic) interventions, such data are very often available through the very Phase 0–IV trials rigorously conducted as part of the regulatory approval process, with a large portion of the data available prior to commercialization. In the case of devices, such data are most often not developed during the regulatory clearance (or approval) processes but are demanded by patients, clinicians, payers, and policymakers nonetheless. Unfortunately the availability of the IGI devices and interventions prior to the conduct of rigorous clinical trials has important impact on trial design and subject accrual (and thus on recruitment strategies). And even if well-designed Pilot and Pivotal trials were conducted for IGI devices, the lack of a graduated paradigm of clinical trials that includes not only the safety and effectiveness of the devices themselves but also the role of the procedural intervention within the context of already existing treatments for the clinical condition, there is insufficient granularity to provide evidence required to guide medical decision-making.

Beyond the differences inherent in or derivative from the dichotomy between the drug/biologic and device regulatory pathways, there are also differences between clinical trials of IGI trials and clinical trials of devices used in surgical (open, nonimage-guided) interventions. Table 3.2 summarizes some of these differences. These differences also affect trial design as will be discussed later in this chapter.

Patent protection for new (not continuation patents) utility or plant patents filed after June 8, 1995, is for 20 years from the date of application and for design patents it is for 14 years from the date on which the patent is granted

Table 3.2 Differences between IGI and traditional non-image guided device clinical trials.

1 Surgical interventions most often include availability of excised tissue, thereby allowing histopathologic evaluation for multiple purposes including, but not limited to, assessment of the underlying preintervention pathology and endpoint determination, thereby necessitating alternative methods for the latter (at least) during IGI trials

2 IGIs are frequently much less invasive and somewhat less costly than are open interventions and therefore often repeatable should the primary result be less durable than desired; hence determination of the time point at which the intervention has been completed may not be readily obvious

3 Adverse events directly related to the IGI tools may not be obvious at the time of the intervention since there is most frequently lack of intraprocedural direct visual observation, thereby necessitating alternative methods for such assessments

(see USPTO for more detail; http://www.uspto.gov/web/offices/pac/mpep/ s2701.html). These periods of protection apply equally for drugs/biologics and devices. However, the period of effective patent protection for devices is much shorter. Devices constantly evolve from one generation to the next. The experience gained and data generated with a device in clinical use form the basis for the development of the device that will be next made available for trial and eventually for clinical deployment. Often these evolved devices may not have sufficient novelty to support new patents or extensions of existing patents. Furthermore, competitors often develop "me-to" devices that are substantively similar to marketed devices while not sufficiently the same to infringe on patent protection. Drugs and biologics generally do not undergo such evolutionary redesign. Instead new generations of drugs and biologics undergo development cycles of much longer durations, are accomplished in conjunction with novel and patentable discovery, and are exclusive of competitors. Given the cost and duration of typical clinical trials for regulatory approval of drugs and biologics, the paradigm used for drug and biologic approvals would not be viable for interventional devices.

There are also important differences in the underlying science for device-based interventions as compared with drugs and biologics, especially the newer generation of "targeted" molecules. Device-based interventions are effective on the basis of biologic and physiologic mechanisms that allow relatively facile "horizontal" translation from one disease state to others, from one clinical utility (as previously defined) to others, from one clinical disease stage to others, and from one anatomic site to others. This is rarely the case for drugs and biologics; and even when "horizontal" translation is possible for systemic therapies, it is generally with far less facility than is the case for device-based interventions. Conducting rigorous clinical trials for device-based interventions across all disease states, clinical utilities, stages of illness, and anatomies using the Phase 0–IV paradigm would be expensive and time consuming and would likely not add value to patient care. Failing to conduct any trials at all to validate proposed horizontal translation is, at the very least, equally indefensible.

Additionally, the human and financial resources of device companies, even the largest, are not equivalent to those of drug and biologic companies. Conducting clinical trials to support the previously described developmental life cycle for device-based interventions would strain the resources of even the largest drug companies, let alone the typical device company, should the clinical trial paradigm used for drug and biologic interventions be demanded for device commercialization, payment, or coverage policy or to support medical decision-making regarding device-based interventions.

Finally, trials of IGIs differ from trials of imaging (e.g., for technology assessment or clinical utilities such as screening, diagnosis, or response assessment) most obviously secondary to the fact that ultimately an IGI trial is a treatment trial with endpoints related to the outcomes of the intervention either on the lesional, organ, or patient level.

3.3 A paradigm for considering IGI clinical trial design

Based on the material provided previously in this chapter, it should be clear that while the Phase 0–IV clinical trial paradigm is workable (albeit with some difficulties in certain circumstances) for trials of drugs and biologics, this paradigm very often needs to be modified for trials of devices. However, the clinical trial paradigm of pilot and pivotal studies to support the commercialization of medical devices in the current regulatory environment is insufficient for the development of data prerequisite to support contemporary medical practice. Furthermore, while novel drugs and biologics often may be initially tested *in vitro* or *ex vivo*, in cell cultures and small animal models, the majority of devices and device-based interventions are tested and optimized in larger animals (if animal models are used at all) with an earlier transition to first-in-human investigations.

The initial studies of IGIs should be designed to focus on device and procedural optimization, improved integration of the IGI "system" (i.e., the interventive device, the imaging tool(s), and the integration of one with the other), establishing appropriate procedural metrics for quality assurance (QA), and developing methods for monitoring the intended and unintended outcomes of the IGI that might appropriately be performed in a variety of anatomic locations, perhaps in related, but different, clinical conditions, but most productively at a single investigational site or perhaps a small number of sites. For example, early evaluation of an ablative device might include performance in the eradication of metastatic lesions to the liver and lung from a variety of primary cancers found in subjects with various stages of disease. Or using Case example 1.3, one might include subjects with primary stage 1 non-small-cell lung cancer (NSCLC) who are going on to surgery so as to optimize the technology toward more complete ablation of the index tumor using a study design commonly referred to as "ablate and resect." Such "early-phase" clinical studies might also serve to establish preliminary safety data at the subject level and evidence of efficacy at a lesional level. While favorable subject-level outcomes will be the ultimate metric for success, understanding the IGI performance at the lesional level is mandatory to provide early "go-no-go" decisions during the development and optimization of the IGI. Similarly, preliminary evidence should be developed to demonstrate that the IGI may be delivered with a sufficient safety margin to support feasibility. Certainly if despite best engineering efforts and expert operator involvement by a physician–scientist there is insufficient evidence of lesional efficacy and subject safety, there would be no reason to proceed to more advanced clinical trials. A trial with the attributes just described would be considered within the description of a Pilot trial using CDRH/FDA nomenclature. For the purposes of this discussion, we classify this type of study as Phase A although there is no such formal paradigm for the classification of device trials.

Assuming success during the aforementioned early-phase trials, subsequent trials might focus on standardizing the performance of the IGI to the extent possible while still allowing for operator intraprocedural judgment, establishing a greater body of evidence to support the safety of the IGI, and beginning to develop evidence of efficacy in expert hands at the lesional and exploratory data of efficacy at the subject (patient) level and in carefully controlled clinical circumstances (i.e., more narrowly defined clinical and anatomic conditions). The measure for efficacy at the lesional level might be clinical and imaging follow-up of the index lesion in some subjects and retaining the ablate and resect model in others. A trial with the attributes described in this paragraph also would be considered within the description of a Pilot trial using CDRH/FDA nomenclature. For the purposes of this discussion, we classify this type of study as Phase B.

Using the Case example 1.3, a study could be designed focusing only on subjects with stage 1 NSCLC treated with radiofrequency ablation (RFA) but using various types of imaging equipment and/or ablation devices in order to standardize technique with the primary aim of establishing safety data and a secondary aim of exploring metrics for efficacy.

Logically the next progression of clinical trial design would confirm the safety and lesional efficacy data developed during the previously performed trials while primarily focusing on estimating the effectiveness of the IGI through a multisite trial with lesional and/or subject-level data likely using historical data for comparison purposes. Using Case example 1.3, this type of study would involve both cancer-specific survival and overall survival as primary aims with secondary aims of safety and local/regional postintervention residual or recurrent disease as well as the rates of retreatment with assisted success. At this stage the trial if rigorously designed might be acceptable as a Pivotal trial (e.g., in studies where subject-level data are used toward the primary aim) but might still be considered a Pilot trial (e.g., in studies where lesional-level data are used toward the primary aim) depending on the details of the study design. For the purposes of this discussion, we classify this type of study as Phase C.

Finally, an IGI might be studied using a multisite trial design with subject-level effectiveness outcome data as the primary endpoint. A randomized clinical trial (RCT) would be the preferred design, but as will be discussed, an RCT may not be feasible or reasonable in some circumstances for a variety of reasons. Such a trial would be considered a Pivotal trial assuming a rigorous design and for the purposes of this discussion is classified as Phase D. Using Case example 1.3, a trial could be designed as an RCT of subjects with inoperable NSCLC (inoperable being defined uniformly as will be discussed later in this chapter) with assignment to receive either RFA, radiotherapy, or the combination of the two. The primary aim would be cancer-specific and overall survival with secondary aims of safety, quality of life (QoL), and cost. The metrics would need to include not only general measures of these outcomes but also measures specific to the anatomic site of the intervention such as pulmonary function. (Again, it must be emphasized that the Phase A–D designations are for discussion purposes only as no such granular clinical trial paradigm exists for IGI trials or any other device-based trials for that matter.)

Table 3.3 Relationship of technology translational stage to clinical trial design typologies.

Stage in translational continuum	Phase 0–IV "equivalent" drug / biologic trial typology*	"Equivalent" FDA device trial typology*	Phase A–D typology as used in text
Basic science discovery/applied engineering concept	Preclinical experiment or Phase 0	Preclinical or Pilot	Preclinical or Phase A
Optimization	Preclinical experiment of Phase 0–IIA	Preclinical or Pilot	Preclinical or Phase A
Feasibility/ standardization/safety/ local biologic effect	Phase I	Pilot	Phase B
Validation for specific applications	Phase II–IV	Pilot	Phase C
Regulatory clearance/ approval	Phase IIB–III	Pilot or Pivotal	Phase C or D
Supportive payer policies promulgated	Phase IIB–IV	Pivotal	Phase C or D
Widespread physician acceptance	Phase IIB–IV	Pivotal	Phase C or D
Patient recognition/ informed demand	Summary of evidence from all sources	Summary of evidence from all sources	Summary of evidence from all sources

*The term "equivalent" is used when citing the drug, biologic, and device typologies since direct equivalency with standard drug and biology clinical trial design (as discussed in Chapter 2) or regulatory device trial design as discussed in this chapter is inappropriate for the reasons discussed in the text.

The previously presented translational continuum might be supported by investigations summarized in Table 3.3, demonstrating the relationship of primary trial "goal" with Phase 0–IV pharma/bio design typology, Pilot–Pivotal device typology, and the Phase A–D typology proposed herein.

Using the aforementioned "shorthand" nomenclature developed for discussion purposes only and not recognized by regulatory agencies, Phase A trials might involve multiple anatomic sites, disease subtypes, and clinical utilities performed at a single investigational site (or a very small number of sites) for the primary purpose of optimizing the intervention and the real-time imaging inherent in the procedure, developing early subject-level safety data, exploring early lesional-level efficacy data, and establishing the quality and performance metrics to be used in subsequent more advanced clinical trial phases presuming success at this level of investigation.

Phase B trials might be performed at a single or small number of investigational sites for the purpose of standardizing the IGI to the extent clinically feasible, developing robust safety data at the subject level coupled with lesional efficacy data and exploratory subject-level efficacy data in a more narrowly defined subject cohort based on specific disease type, clinical utility, and limited anatomic locations appropriate to the disease type and clinical utility under investigation.

Phase C trials would likely be multisite studies to confirm the previously obtained safety data and the previously established lesional efficacy data with translation to effectiveness data at both lesional and subject levels. Again, the inclusion and exclusion criteria would result in a more narrowly defined definition so as to allow translation from the trial cohort to an appropriate clinical setting.

Phase D trials would be multisite studies focused on effectiveness with comparison to alternative interventions using RCTs when possible and alternative trial designs where RCTs are not feasible or reasonable. Note that Phase C and D trials could be designed as Pivotal trials to support FDA approval if sufficiently robust.

We suggest that the trialist designing a clinical trial of an IGI first carefully consider the maturity of the IGI of interest (based on the parameters of disease state and stage, clinical utility, and anatomic site) and the appropriate goal(s) of the trial being designed given existing data relative to the aforementioned parameters. The trialist together with the protocol development team should then decide what phase trial (A–D) is most appropriate before proceeding with the task of developing the protocol and determining the study design. In some cases, the Phase 0–IV paradigm does work for device clinical trials with minor modification, and in such cases the trialist is advised to utilize the classification system described in Chapter 2 with modifications as required—recognizing that the CDRH/FDA does not formally recognize that trial classification scheme.

Radiotherapy trials, including those radiotherapy trials that evaluate radiotherapy in conjunction with systemic therapies (drugs and/or biologics) and/or surgery and/or other types of IGIs, are a particular case in which the paradigm of Phase I–IV clinical trials has been adapted quite successfully.

Many radiotherapy interventions are not IGIs as defined herein as those interventions do not involve imaging for real-time guidance, monitoring, and/or endpoint determination. Instead these radiotherapy interventions might use imaging for procedural planning much as open surgical procedures do. However, increasingly radiotherapy interventions are integrating imaging during the real-time performance of the intervention and therefore are IGIs. Finally, since nearly all radiotherapy interventions are local–regional interventions using devices, there are many similarities with IGIs as described herein; and trials of radiotherapy interventions also have many similarities with IGI trials. To follow we discuss specific considerations of radiotherapy clinical trials.

3.4 Radiotherapy trials

The basics of therapeutic trials as well as the definitions of Phase I, II, and III studies are described in Chapter 2. In this section, we describe the additional considerations needed for the design and conduct of clinical trials with radiotherapy. These principles apply to radiotherapy-alone trials or radiotherapy in combination with other modalities such as chemotherapy or surgery. There are several challenges in the design of radiation interventional trials. First, late effects from radiotherapy often occur months to years after the delivery of treatment, which means that the intervals of observation necessary in a clinical study to determine if a regimen is safe may not be feasible. Second, many clinical trials in the past, particularly in the Phase II setting, have been performed in unselected patient populations, which is an expensive and inefficient approach. Biomarker- or mechanistically directed clinical trials in appropriately selected patient populations are needed to address this challenge. Third, many experimental radiotherapy regimens are introduced in the curative setting of cancer care, and therefore the ethics of these trials must be carefully considered.

3.4.1 Preclinical radiotherapy studies

All trials of radiotherapy whether of radiation alone or in combination with other modalities should be based upon the biological principles underlying the effects of radiation on tumor and normal tissues [3, 4]. This requires an understanding of the basic concepts of radiation biology as well as preclinical studies that support the science of the proposed trial. Preclinical studies are particularly important in trials of radiation and drugs because of toxicity concerns [3, 5]. Preclinical studies should involve clinically relevant regimens and not only evaluate acute and late toxicities of therapeutic approaches but should also investigate the optimal dosing and schedule of agents to maximize response, thus enhancing the therapeutic ratio of the experimental regimen. Importantly, these studies should also attempt to determine the mechanism for the enhanced therapeutic ratio as well as identify targets of such mechanisms. Mechanistic studies and identification of targets will greatly enhance the design of a radiation clinical trial and assist in the identification of companion biomarkers.

3.4.2 Phase I radiotherapy studies

The primary objective of a Phase I radiotherapy trial is similar to Phase I drug studies: the evaluation of safety of the experimental regimen. The primary endpoint is typically the assessment of toxicity and safety and identification of the recommended Phase II dose. Secondary endpoints should be considered including a preliminary assessment of clinical outcome and exploratory studies of biomarkers. The design and application of a Phase I radiotherapy trial may be different from drug studies [6]. In general, Phase I radiotherapy data are generated from studies that are cancer or site specific. This is because the assessment of toxicities and safety (the primary endpoint of a Phase I study) when administering radiation is related to the region where the radiotherapy is delivered and the dose and fractionation schedule used. Radiation-related toxicities are either *acute*, those that occur during or immediately after the delivery of radiotherapy, or *late*, those that occur months to years after the delivery of radiotherapy. These toxicities are related to the normal tissues exposed to radiation. For example, the spectrum of acute toxicities when treating the pelvis with radiation may include diarrhea, skin redness or breakdown, and cytopenias, whereas the acute toxicities when treating the thorax may include esophagitis and skin redness. Therefore, the tolerance of a radiotherapy regimen might be dependent upon the location treated, and therefore, Phase I studies are usually restricted to one site or tumor type. In addition, the spectrum of toxicities (particularly late toxicities) may be different between a palliative and curative radiotherapy regimen. Given the typical long-term goal of developing experimental approaches for improving cure rates, usually Phase I studies are performed in the curative setting. These considerations represent important differences between radiotherapy and drug-alone Phase I studies.

It is important to think about the next step in the development of the experimental regimen when designing the Phase I study. Questions to consider are as follows:

1 What setting, palliative or curative, is appropriate for the experimental regimen?
2 What is the standard therapy for the tumor site being treated?
3 What is the role of conventional therapies such as chemotherapy or surgery?
4 How should conventional therapies, if appropriate, be integrated into an experimental regimen?
5 What are the appropriate biomarkers to evaluate?
6 How can a Phase II study with an unselected patient population be avoided?

As mentioned above, Phase I studies are typically performed in patients undergoing curative radiotherapy [7–10]. This raises ethical considerations because an experimental approach is being added to a potentially curative treatment regimen requiring a multidisciplinary discussion of the proposed study. However, total dose and fractionation differ between curative and palliative treatment regimens. Therefore, an experimental approach that is evaluated in the Phase I setting using a palliative radiotherapy regimen cannot automatically be used in the curative setting for Phase II or III studies. If a palliative radiotherapy regimen is selected for a Phase I study [11] and the long-term goal is to develop the experimental approach for the curative setting, additional safety data must be collected with a curative radiotherapy regimen prior to moving to a Phase II or III study.

The determination of the palliative or curative setting for the Phase I study guides the role of standard treatments in the study including the use of conventional therapies such as surgery and chemotherapy. One approach for Phase I studies of radiotherapy with newer chemotherapeutic agents such as targeted therapies is in the preoperative or neoadjuvant setting [10, 12]. For example, standard therapy for rectal cancer patients is often chemotherapy with radiation delivered over 5 weeks followed by surgical resection and additional chemotherapy. An experimental agent can be added to the standard neoadjuvant chemotherapy and radiation regimen followed by surgery. There are several advantages of this approach including assessment of pathological response to therapy in the surgical specimen and incorporation of imaging and tissue biomarkers that can be evaluated before, during, and after the standard therapies [13].

Regardless of whether a neoadjuvant setting is considered for a radiotherapy Phase I trial, strong consideration should be made for the incorporation of biomarkers and particularly imaging biomarkers. The selection of appropriate biomarkers is guided by the preclinical data and knowledge of the mechanism of action of the experimental approach. Biomarker evaluation in Phase I studies is exploratory only and therefore can be used to generate hypotheses for the Phase II setting.

If a new chemotherapeutic agent is being added to a radiotherapy regimen, single-agent safety and pharmacokinetic and pharmacodynamic data from human studies of the agent alone are helpful in the design of the radiation and experimental agent Phase I study. Single-agent safety data may be used to guide decisions regarding the appropriate location of radiotherapy delivery. For example, if diarrhea is a major side effect of the agent alone, treatment of a pelvic malignancy in the trial may not be wise because of concerns for overlapping toxicities. The schedule of agent delivery and the pharmacodynamic effect of the agent are also useful in study design. In general, a regimen that allows for exposure of the tumor to drug during as many fractions of radiation as possible is preferred. When single-agent drug data are known, a limited dose escalation design is typically used. A common approach is to select a dose of the drug that is one or two levels below the maximum tolerated dose (MTD) identified in the drug-alone Phase I study. Therefore only 1–3 drug dose escalation levels are incorporated into the study design. Another approach is to consider using full-dose standard chemotherapeutic agents and escalate radiation doses [14].

One additional consideration when adding a new agent to a standard radiotherapy or chemoradiotherapy regimen is the use of a lead-in of the experimental agent alone prior to the standard treatment [9, 13]. This allows for an independent assessment of toxicity as well as evaluation of the effect of the agent alone on any biomarker that is being explored as a secondary endpoint in the trial.

For either a radiotherapy alone or radiotherapy and drug combination Phase I study, standard Phase I dose escalation rules and MTD definitions are used (described in Chapter 2). The definition of dose-limiting toxicities (DLT) may differ, however, from drug-alone studies. Most trials should start with DLT definition of any Grade IV hematologic or Grade III nonhematologic toxicity that is definitely, probably, or possibly related to the experimental regimen. However, exceptions to these rules should be considered and incorporated into the DLT rules. For example, treatment of the pelvis with standard chemotherapy and radiation for pelvic cancer commonly causes Grade III diarrhea. One exception to the DLT rules that could be incorporated is "Grade III diarrhea that is not controlled with antidiarrheal agents" or "only Grade IV diarrhea." Additional DLT rules that should be considered are (i) any break of radiotherapy of one week or longer, (ii) inability to deliver standard therapy, and (iii) surgical morbidity.

Toxicity assessment for the determination of DLT is typically scored during the entire standard treatment regimen—weekly during a course of radiotherapy and for 30–90 days after the completion of radiotherapy regimen. For dose escalation, radiotherapy-alone studies' toxicity is usually scored for the time period (6–24 months) when late effects may appear. This approach, of course, increases substantially the duration of the study. After the selected toxicity scoring period is passed and no DLTs are identified, dose escalation to the next dose level may proceed in a similar fashion to drug-alone Phase I studies. Identification of late toxicities in Phase I radiotherapy trials is a major challenge to study design [5, 6]. There are certainly practical and time limitations as described. In addition, there are clinical difficulties in identifying late toxicities and distinguishing these from tumor recurrence and other posttreatment toxicities. Some investigators have advocated alternative approaches to assessment of late effects such as TITE-CRM methodologies [6]. Regardless of the approach used and time period employed for DLT assessment, patients on Phase I radiotherapy studies should be followed and toxicity determined for at least 1 year after the completion of radiation.

One final consideration for Phase I radiotherapy regimens is to incorporate an expanded subject cohort at the identified MTD. This approach will permit a preliminary assessment of efficacy as well as allow for a more precise evaluation of biomarkers.

3.4.3 Phase II/III radiotherapy studies

The decision to proceed with a Phase II radiotherapy alone or radiotherapy and chemotherapy combination study is dependent upon the determination of safety, the preliminary assessment of efficacy, and the exploratory evaluation of biomarkers. This is a complicated, important decision. Phase II studies as described in Chapter 2 are usually larger, have significant ethical considerations particularly if employed in the curative setting, and may require the expenditure of greater resources compared to Phase I studies.

The primary endpoint of a Phase II trial is usually a measure of efficacy of the experimental regimen. Secondary endpoints include additional assessment of toxicity and biomarker evaluation. Consideration should be made for selection of subjects based upon the mechanism of action of the agent or the results of biomarker studies. For example, if a targeted agent is to be used in the study, expression of the target in tumor may be required for study entry. Such an approach "enriches" the subject population with those patients who are expected to respond to the experimental approach based upon prior clinical experience, the results of the Phase I study or the results of drug-alone studies.

The selection of the appropriate efficacy endpoint is particularly important in Phase II radiotherapy studies. Response rate is often not helpful because of delayed time to response to radiotherapy, residual unevaluable masses versus scarring after radiotherapy, the development of progressive disease outside of the radiotherapy field, and the underlying high local response rates to radiotherapy. A validated efficacy endpoint must be chosen; examples include pathological response rate, local or locoregional control rates, locoregional time to progression, and survival. The efficacy endpoint will also depend upon the tumor being treated and the current standard therapy employed for that tumor.

Continued collection of additional toxicity data for both acute and late toxicities is essential to confirm the safety of the experimental regimen. Early stopping rules for toxicity should be considered (see Chapter 7). The collection of late toxicity data in the larger group of subjects within a Phase II study will be helpful in the design of a Phase III study.

3.5 Caveats in the design and conduct of IGI trials

Once an appropriate phase trial is determined, study design may then begin. In so doing, we suggest further consideration of the following caveats and pitfalls. The first among these is the common pitfall of overreaching during the design of the trial. Often trialists are determined to design and conduct a trial at a more advanced phase than can be justified on the basis of existing data and previous clinical trials. This scenario is most often secondary to the fact that many IGI devices may be in common clinical use despite the absence of rigorous data, justifying that use for a particular clinical purpose. Understanding the difference between clinical practice and clinical science is an important point when designing a clinical trial. It is important that the protocol development team spend some time on rigorous critique of their work to ensure that the study designed can be justified to potential sponsors, ethics committees, and the referral base, as well as to ensure robust recruitment.

For example, again turning to the hypothetical clinical trial proposed in Chapter 1 (Case example 1.3), the protocol development team needs to consider if there are sufficient preliminary data to allow an RCT among RFA, radiotherapy, and combination therapy in general. If so, has there been sufficient standardization to allow the use of multiple types of RFA generators, applicators, from various vendors? Has there been sufficient standardization to determine the exact protocol by which combination therapy will be delivered, such as the order of interventions, the time between the first and second intervention, and any dose adjustment in the radiotherapy when delivered in conjunction with RFA rather than as the sole intervention? If these matters have not been explored and defined, more basic clinical trials are more appropriate and prerequisite to a large RCT.

3.5.1 Defining the clinical trial cohort
The cohort(s) to be recruited into the clinical trial should be composed on the basis of inclusion and exclusion criteria that are translatable to clinical practice so that the results of the trial will result in clinically useful information. To that end, it is important that the cohort is defined in a way that results in cohort homogeneity. The cohort inclusion criteria should therefore define the disease, stage, lesion characteristics, and when appropriate subject criteria such as functional status, degree of impairment, and comorbidities (appropriate for the phase of study contemplated by the study design).

Vague characteristics that are open to interpretation should be avoided—in particular the term "not a surgical candidate" that is often used to "define" IGI trial eligibility should be avoided. Instead, eligibility could be defined by the underlying reason that the subject is not a surgical candidate. There may be a significant variability in subject characteristics that might contribute to a person being classified as "not a surgical candidate" ranging from patient personal preference, operator personal preference, chronic comorbidities of a particular severity level, advanced stage of the target disease, previous therapeutic intervention complicating the potential operative field, or a concurrent acute illness or acute complicating condition. It is important to specify which of these (or others not listed herein) reasons are the exact inclusionary or exclusionary criteria used in the trial in order to allow the clinical trial results to be interpreted accurately.

In Case example 1.3, the definition of an inoperable lesion is critical. The impact of RFA, radiotherapy, and the combination of the two is quite different in a subject who has baseline compromised pulmonary function tests as compared with a subject who simply does not choose to undergo surgery although physiologically able to have such surgery. Furthermore, the threshold for performing surgery in people with pulmonary compromise is quite different among surgeons and institutions. Therefore, defined measurable thresholds are necessary when constructing a multi-institutional trial as compared with a single-site study.

Another useful definition of the clinical cohort for the trial is by identifying subjects on the basis of a particular upcoming medical decision point, leading to a "standard of care" treatment option for which the subjects might otherwise be considered eligible. For example, subjects might be considered eligible for the IGI trial if they would be considered candidates for an open surgical intervention that is otherwise considered the usual option for the clinical condition under investigation. This is an especially valuable method of defining the trial cohort if the results of the trial are to be compared with one or more historical datasets derived from previous clinical trials of that specific surgical intervention in the same clinical condition.

Just as is true in early-phase trials of drugs and biologics, consideration should be given to defining the subject cohort so as to focus on subjects with advanced disease states with few viable standard of care treatment options. However, the trialist should recognize that these patients may be particularly vulnerable, especially if the principal investigator also is the treating physician. Therefore, the investigational procedure should not be positioned as one offering great hope, but instead the subjects should understand that their enrollment in the study is based on their goodwill and willingness to contribute to the advancement of science rather than the hope of a potential benefit.

Equally important as defining the subject cohort is the definition of the control group. The constitution of the control group will be determined by the phase of the study and the trial primary and secondary aims and endpoints. In many early-phase device trials there will be no control group (historical or prospective). However, should a control group be necessary based on the study design, carefully specifying the constitution of the control cohort is critical. The chapters in this text dealing with study design will cover the attributes of various control group options.

3.5.2 Standardization of the study procedures and quality assurance

Systemic pharmacotherapies and biologic interventions generally have fixed administration protocols based on one of several physiologic parameters (e.g., dose per body surface area or dose per body mass, etc.). The fixed administration protocol may escalate during dose-ranging studies (typically Phase I), but in more advanced trials one dose or a small number of doses are used for all subjects. The timing of the administration is also most often mandated for all subjects. Even modifications of the dose for individual participants, including withholding one or several cycles, are carefully prescribed in advance based on set criteria. There is very limited, if any, protocol variation left to the investigators' discretion in trials of systemic interventions.

IGIs, as is also true for open surgical interventions, include the potential for operator variations during procedure performance and often for very good reason. However, the need for operator judgment during performance of the investigational and (if one is included in the study design) the reference standard of care procedure must be balanced against the need for standardization to the extent possible. The protocol development team should specify any and all features of the procedure(s) that might potentially impact the outcome variables being assessed. In addition to cohort characteristics that should be specified for IGI trials that are similar to those usually specified for system intervention trials, details that might be specified could include, but are not limited to:

1 The characteristics of the index lesion(s) to be targeted.
2 The number of such lesions per organ and/or per subject.
3 The location of such lesions per organ and/or per subject.
4 The type (and potentially manufacturer and model) of device(s) used (based on relative equivalency among the options based on parameters important to the outcome measures being assessed).
5 The imaging modality(ies) that should be used for targeting the lesion(s), for monitoring the intervention, and for assessing the procedural endpoint—these could all be the same modality or could be different modalities for each purpose.
6 The manner in which subjects should be monitored through the pre-, intra-, and postprocedural time periods.
7 The precise manner in which the interventive devices are to be used throughout the IGI procedure.
8 The exact data that are to be collected to document all of the above.

Aspects of procedure performance that have no potential for affecting the outcome measures being collected should not be overly specified. Doing so contributes to the potential of protocol deviations and violations, thereby undermining the credibility of the results. However, procedure performance characteristics that definitely will affect outcome measures or that might conceivably affect outcome measures should be specified in sufficient detail to eliminate or minimize such impact. Specifying and monitoring adherence to the clinical trial operator performance characteristics is always important, but becomes even more critical during multisite and/or multioperator clinical trials. Many operators may have used the IGI device(s) and imaging modality(ies) for the same or similar clinical conditions outside the trial setting. Many will have strong preferences as to how the procedure should be performed. It is important when participating in a clinical trial that personal preference takes a "backseat" to the specified performance characteristics that are mandated by trial design. Including important collaborators knowledgeable in the intervention(s) included in the trail as members of the protocol development team is essential to achieving consensus around the protocol details. However, once those details have been determined, operators who are not willing or able to follow the protocol as written should decline participation rather than participating while contributing deviations, violations, and invalid data.

In the hypothetical trial defined as Case example 1.3, all the subjects must be eligible for either RFA or radiotherapy using the precise protocol, technique, and equipment as defined. If the various physician-scientists cannot agree on these characteristics and follow them precisely, the trial will either be infeasible or there will be too many protocol deviations/violations to allow valid analyses.

It may be useful to define areas in which operator variability is allowable and indeed encouraged along with clinical determinants to assist with choices among allowable options. In short, the difference between allowable real-time medical decision-making and off-protocol actions should be defined and recognized. To this end protocol initiation meetings and periodic investigator meetings are quite useful as is a rigorous QA program.

3.5.3 IGI trial QA

QA for an IGI trial begins well before the protocol is initiated and indeed should be included in the trial design. First, there should be a rigorous site and operator qualification program that might include an educational component, mentoring, and proctored procedures. Additionally, it might be useful to require that results of the first several (exact number to be determined) cases are reviewed by a QA committee individually before the next case is recruited.

Second, there should be a rigorous procedural QA program defined in the protocol that includes the exact data elements to be collected during the pre-, intra-, and postprocedural time periods. These data elements may include subject-specific data (such as vital signs, medications, and/or other physical, biological, and physiologic measures), device-specific operation characteristics (such as balloon inflation pressures and times, ablation temperature measurements, and infusion rates and times), and critical imaging modality capture at predefined procedural time points.

Third, there should be imaging QA that in many ways will be similar to the requirements of non-IGI imaging trials. These QA elements might include site prequalification based on equipment and personnel training and experience. In addition, there might be ongoing QA based on submitted image data and/or periodic site visits.

3.5.4 IGI clinical trial endpoints: measures of success and failure

There are several issues related to defining success and failure that must be addressed. The first of these is recognizing that IGI procedures (as is true for many other types of interventions) are measured by success or lack thereof (along a continuum from completely successful through some measure of partial success to complete failure) as well as complicated by unintended adverse event(s) or not. The degree of success may to large extent be unrelated to the presence or absence of adverse events. Hence, a completely successful procedure as measured by the primary endpoints of that outcome could occur without any adverse event or might occur in the context of adverse events from minor (Grade 1) through lethal adverse events (Grade 5). Therefore, the composite outcome of the trial must take into account both metrics of success and adverse events, especially when comparison is made to historical or prospective data reflecting alternative interventional outcomes.

Second, as stated previously, minimally or noninvasive IGIs may often be repeated to treat residual disease or recurrent disease at the site of initial intervention or to treat new disease not within the initial field of primary intervention. A repeated intervention may even be a part of the initial intent to treat plan (considered as a staged intervention). Since several important and frequent outcomes of investigational interventions are time based (e.g., time to progression, survival statistics, 30-day mortality and morbidity rates), it is important to define the time of the intervention as the point from which these time-based outcomes are measured. It is inappropriate to assume the date of the initial intervention as "time 0" for all types of interventions, for all clinical utilities, and for all disease states. It is equally inappropriate to allow an infinite number of repeated interventions as part of the protocol either (i) with a reset of "time 0" to the most recent intervention or (ii) with retention of "time 0" as the date of the initial intervention. Either of these latter two strategies has significant implications toward interpretation of trial results.

Instead, it is suggested to consider during design of the trial whether or not repeated interventions should sensibly be allowed based on the disease state, clinical utility, and the mechanism of action of the intervention. If repeated interventions are to be allowed as part of the protocol, the number of repeated interventions and the time period during which the interventions may be repeated should be specified. As well, the acceptable reasons for repeated interventions (e.g., staged procedure plan as intent to treat, residual disease on early postprocedure assessment, recurrent disease on later postprocedure assessment, new disease outside of the initial treatment field) should be clearly stated. Finally, the trial design should address how repeated interventions outside of the protocol stipulations are to be managed (e.g., censure, treatment failure, or variably based on the reason for the off-protocol intervention).

Additionally, consideration should be given to paradigm of measuring success and failure similar to the criteria applied to studies of endovascular intervention in peripheral vascular disease as summarized in Table 3.4.

Table 3.4 Measuring success and failure in IGI trials.

Primary-Assisted Success—Result of intervention including repeated interventions outside of the initial field of intervention to assist with the primary outcome (but no repeated interventions within the initial field of intervention)

Secondary-Assisted Success—Result of intervention including repeated interventions within the initial field of intervention to assist with the primary outcome

Failure—Residual, recurrent, or new disease leading to failure to achieve the primary outcome measure for success (subject refuses or is ineligible for additional intervention, dies with disease, or otherwise fails to achieve the primary outcome measure for success).

As previously stated, the decisions as to whether or not additional intervention events should be included within the protocol and as to how and when to measure success should take into consideration the proposed utility of the intervention and whether the outcome will be measured at the lesional, organ, or subject level. In early-phase studies, the success or failure of an IGI at the lesional level may be assessed by comparison with pathology in a trial that includes resection of the lesion to which the IGI was applied.

Finally, there is the issue of how success is measured. In many circumstances clinical metrics are the most appropriate measure of success. For example, in some cases disease-specific or overall survival is most appropriate. In other cases severity of symptoms, measured by pain or quality-of-life scales, for example, may be appropriate. However, in many circumstances imaging is used for response assessment. Imaging is frequently used for response assessment in a variety of disease states and for a variety of interventions. However, imaging response assessment criteria must be validated for specific disease states and for specific types of interventions. For example, the Response Evaluation Criteria in Solid Tumors (RECIST) and the PET Response Criteria in Solid Tumors (PERCIST) are often used for assessment response of tumor burden to systemic interventions by drugs and biologics [15, 16]. However, these criteria are not applicable to response assessment of oncologic IGIs unless significantly modified. For example, immediate postablation lesion size (uni- or bidimensional or volumetric) is generally larger than baseline measurement for thermal and cryotherapies. Many types of transvascular cancer embolotherapies also demonstrate postprocedural imaging findings that would complicate evaluation using either of these two response assessment criteria. However, the postprocedural lesion size and metabolic activity measurements reflect not only the underlying tumor but also the effects of the intervention. Furthermore, recurrent or residual disease often does not present as enlargement of the baseline tumor size, nor does it present as new or increased metabolic activity as compared with baseline when oncologic IGIs are used. In recognition of these facts, there have been modified imaging response criteria proposed for some oncologic IGI response assessment such as the European Association for the Study of Liver (EASL) modification of WHO size criteria or mRECIST for hepatic IGI in hepatocellular carcinoma [17, 18].

In specific disease states and IGI types for which validated imaging response criteria exist, these could be employed in the proposed clinical trial design. However, if this is not the case, initial use of imaging response criteria should be exploratory only with the purpose of validating the criteria for use in subsequent trials. Validation could be on the basis of pathology (e.g., ablate and resect trial, or clinical outcome correlation, or both). The validation of imaging response criteria could be a secondary or exploratory aim of Phase A or B studies that are primarily focused on optimization of the intervention and/or metrics of safety. By so doing, the validated imaging response criteria could be available for subsequent Phase C and D studies.

As previously noted, a key difference between IGIs and nonimaging-guided open surgical procedures is the lack of tissue confirmation after minimally or non-invasive therapies. By way of example, in oncologic IGI there is no equivalent evidence of a surgical tumor-free margin as would be the case after surgical excision. An important advancement yet to be achieved is discovering and validating such a noninvasive metric, perhaps using a fused dataset derived from multiparametric analysis employing tissue and imaging biomarkers.

3.6 Potential impediments to the design and conduct of IGI clinical trials

There are several potential impediments to the design and conduct of IGI clinical trials. However, there are also potential strategies to overcome them.

3.6.1 Evaluation of the placebo effect

When attempting to evaluate the contribution of placebo effect, one might consider a trial design in which subjects are randomized between receiving the investigational IGI and a sham procedure. When the IGI is a noninvasive modality (e.g., MRI-guided focused ultrasound surgery (MRgFUS) or externally administered radiation therapy), this study design is very possible and has indeed been used [19]. The design may also incorporate crossover for subjects assigned to the sham arm who have continued indications for intervention after completing the defined postintervention follow-up period. However, when the investigational IGI is a transvascular, endoluminal, or percutaneous procedure that involves risk of anesthesia (usually conscious sedation) and the invasive access procedure, it is difficult to justify randomization to a sham procedure. This clinical trial design issue is similar to what might be encountered in studies of surgical procedures. Therefore alternative study designs should be considered and may draw from the surgical clinical trial design experience. One design option might include the investigational IGI in both arms, one in conjunction with a standard of care therapy and the other without the standard of care therapy. Another might evaluate an investigational IGI in comparison with a standard of care IGI or other local–regional therapy.

3.6.2 Masking or blinding of investigators

An important source of bias in the conduct of clinical trials is investigator preference for or against the investigational intervention. Masking or blinding of the investigatory team to the subjects' assignments to the investigational or the control group(s) is one method of avoiding this type of bias. However, it is most often not possible to mask the investigator(s) performing the intervention (the operator of either the investigational or control procedure) as to any particular subject's assignment. Therefore, it is not possible to completely avoid this type of bias. This impediment is similar to what might be encountered when designing surgical or invasive cardiology clinical trials. However, the impact of this bias can be significantly reduced by arranging for a masked or blinded group of investigators to perform all of the pre-, intra-, and postprocedural evaluations and data collection. This group of investigators should not perform any of the investigational or control procedures. Data collection forms that might identify the type of procedure performed should not be shared with these evaluators.

3.6.3 Impediments related to "standard of care" control interventions

As is true in other treatment trials, there may not be a universally acknowledged standard of care treatment to which the investigational IGI can be compared. In fact, the standard of care may be legitimately debated among experts in the field. A variant of this impediment is the scenario in which there is active and ongoing research related to treatment alternatives for the targeted disease state. As a result, the acknowledged standard of care may change, sometimes more than once, during the time period during which the IGI trial will be conducted. Comparing the investigational IGI to a treatment not acknowledged as the then current standard of care may discredit the results of the IGI trial. Strategies to overcome this impediment include (i) allowing the standard of care in the control group to vary over time but still insisting on a single comparator at any given time, or (ii) using random assignment to multiple comparison groups within the control arm, or (iii) allowing the participating sites to choose among a preselected set of standard of care therapies in a "fielder's choice" design. Each of these options carries with it downsides and biases that may be corrected with varying degrees of success. Each of these options will also likely mandate an increase in the sample size of the study, entirely due to the increase in sample size of the control group. While not an option that is easily embraced, it may be necessary to delay the implementation of the IGI trial until after there is greater agreement as to the treatment to be used as the control. As will be discussed shortly, if all other strategies have been explored and are not viable, a study design that does not involve a concurrent control group may be considered in this circumstance. For example, a single-arm study with comparison to both historical controls and "hypothetical" best expected outcome from among the available and still in study alternatives might be a useful trial design as a placeholder. Such a study would develop statistically valid safety and efficacy/effectiveness outcomes that could be used in the future to design a randomized trial or might have to be used as the best clinical evidence available given the state of the art at the time.

3.6.4 Rapid evolution of the IGI device and related devices: multiple similar competitive IGI devices

As has been previously discussed, IGI devices (unlike drugs and biologic agents) are evolving such that the current devices used in clinical care also serve as prototypes for new devices. The life cycle of medical devices used in IGIs is such that the device(s) included in a clinical trial may be obsolete prior to the conclusion of the trial and publication of the results. As has been previously discussed, there may be multiple similar IGI devices that are marketed by the same or competitor vendors that all may be used for the same purpose. We have previously described the need to limit the number of variables in a clinical trial. In the circumstance of multiple similar or evolving devices, the need to limit variables may preclude using all the available devices within the clinical trial. In addition when a particular vendor sponsors or funds a trial, that vendor may have little or no interest in including devices from its competitors within the trial. Again, as has been previously discussed, the ability of device companies or federal and philanthropic funding sources to support multiple similar trials differentiated only by the particular make and model of device employed is very limited and probably appropriate. Therefore, early in the design of the IGI trial, it must be determined whether the trial will employ multiple devices or only a single device and, if the former, whether or not that decision will mandate an increase in the sample size and therefore the cost of the trial. If the trial is to be implemented as a single device trial, thought should also be given to when and how to determine the translatability of the results among the similar devices in the category. The regulatory aspect of this issue is beyond the scope of the chapter.

3.6.5 The feasibility of RCTs of IGIs

RCTs are not appropriate for early-phase clinical trials, whether of drugs, biologics, or devices. However, traditionally RCTs have been viewed as lingua franca for later phase (Phase III and IV) trials of drugs and biologics in most cases. Trialists dedicated to investigating IGIs should aspire to a similar standard. In some cases, pursuing an RCT of an IGI may be difficult but still possible, and when this is the case, unless there are overwhelming reasons to the contrary, an RCT should be used. However, there are circumstances, some of which have already been discussed in this chapter, that make RCTs infeasible for IGIs. Some reasons that might make an RCT infeasible, which have not yet been discussed, include the following. First, the alternative treatments may be offered by competing clinical services, each with a vested interest in the status quo. Such differences should not preclude an RCT in theory, but in practice they often do. In such circumstances, it is suggested that an intermediate step be undertaken: conducting a trial using an alternative design with the plan to conduct an RCT at some later date when sufficient evidence derived by other designs is available to convince individuals with potentially competing interests to collaborate.

Second, there may be a lack of alternative treatments to which the IGI may be compared for a variety of clinical conditions. In such cases, while the IGI could be compared to no treatment at all, this may raise ethical issues especially if the IGI is available as standard of care outside of the clinical trial. In such cases, it is suggested that an alternative trial design is implemented rather than having no rigorously developed evidence at all.

Third, as has been previously stated, the 510(k) regulatory pathway (and some would argue even the PMA pathway that does demand IDE-supported trials) allows devices to come to market without rigorous RCTs that demonstrate clinical effectiveness in comparison with alternative interventions. Therefore in many, indeed most circumstances the IGI being investigated is available as standard of care outside of the clinical trial. Practically, it becomes very difficult to randomize subjects to the arm that does not get the IGI, especially if there are clinical biases on the part of patients, patient families, and referring clinicians. Paradoxically, it is often the very physicians who demand evidence for IGIs developed by RCTs who refuse to allow their patients to become subjects in an RCT of such IGIs. In such cases, it is strongly advised to consider alternative study designs even for later phase trials rather than forego the availability of data-driven evidence at all.

Fourth, there are valid circumstances in which an RCT is simply not ethical [20]. Such circumstances include the lack of availability of an alternative treatment as standard of care or strong evidence that available alternatives are severely lacking in benefit or have significant associated adverse events. That said, the temptation to simply give up on an RCT design prematurely should be avoided. Using an alternative trial design should be undertaken only if and when a critical evaluation of implementing an RCT determines that such a trial is not possible. This determination should include input by "disinterested" members of the protocol development team.

3.6.6 Impediments to and pitfalls in the conduct of the trial

Whatever trial design is chosen and then implemented, there are practical impediments to and pitfalls in the conduct of a clinical trial. Many of these are in common with trials of other types of therapies and include, but are not limited to, issues such as retention of subjects for the expected duration of participation once accrued, ensuring completeness and integrity of data collected during the duration of participation, and avoidance of protocol deviations and violations. The latter of these issues has already been discussed in relation to the difference between allowed operator decision-making (per the protocol) and variations that fall outside of such allowed operator decision-making.

The trialist is advised to set realistic accrual goals that include a ramp-up at the time of trial initiation at each participating site. These accrual goals should take into account the previously discussed impediments such as "turf," subject, family, referring physician preferences, and competing interventions (including the investigational intervention available off trial). However, the trial should also include an accrual monitoring plan with periodic assessments as to actual accrual as compared with planned accrual. At each of these assessment time points, it is advised that the PI, with input from the DSMB or steering committee, make a determination as to what opportunities for improvement exist should accrual be lacking. The protocol may need to be modified with regard to inclusion and exclusion criteria, description of the included tests and procedures, or the intensity of follow-up if any or all of these are believed to be impediments to accrual.

Along with monitoring accrual, the study design should include a plan to deal with adverse events that should define severity, relatedness, and expectedness. Members of the study team other than the operator or others with perceived bias or conflict of interest should perform possible the determination of these three attributes for each adverse event. The assessment should use a commonly understood severity and classification scale such as the National Cancer Institute Common Terminology Criteria for Adverse Events (NCI CTCAE) at the most current version (http://ctep.cancer.gov/protocolDevelopment/electronic_applications/ctc.htm#ctc_40). This tool is very useful for nononcologic disease states and interventions. There are very few IGI-related adverse events that cannot be accommodated by this tool, but so few that the tool should be considered more often than not. Expected adverse events should be defined prior to the outset of the trial and may be classified as likely, unlikely but still possible, and rare. Relatedness is often classified using a five-point scale such as (i) definitely related, (ii) likely related, (iii) indeterminate as to relationship, (iv) likely unrelated, and (v) definitely unrelated. Reports to the oversight bodies (local IRBs, central IRB, DSMB, sponsor, etc.) may then be made uniformly using a standardized nomenclature and rating system.

3.7 Special considerations and the future

Clinical trials of investigational IGIs may be complicated by factors including, but not limited to, such examples as an:

1 IGI used in conjunction with other systemic (drug or biologic) and/or local–regional (surgery, radiation therapy) interventions
2 IGI used in conjunction with another IGI
3 IGI compared with another IGI

These circumstances are further complicated when one or more of the interventions used in combination or as comparators have not been previously validated with rigor. Unfortunately, this scenario is not at all infrequent. Therefore, it is incumbent on the protocol development team to critically evaluate such special circumstances early in the discussion of trial design to ensure that alternatives are considered.

Special consideration must also be given to IGI trials (or any other type of trial for that matter) that have multiple purposes such as the combination of a scientific goal with the goal of achieving regulatory approval from the FDA or garnering coverage or payment policy support from a payer such as CMS (for Medicare or

Medicaid). In such cases, it is advised to consult with the appropriate agency(ies) regarding the proposed trial design well in advance so as to incorporate their feedback and potentially their approval.

3.7.1 Conclusion

The future for minimally and noninvasive IGI in a variety of disease states and clinical conditions is bright. The paradigm of evidence-based medicine is becoming more predominant. The development of such evidence through clinical trials of various designs is critical to the continued and improved availability of IGIs. Interventions will likely be targeted by information beyond purely anatomic imaging that is most frequently used today. Therefore, functional and molecular data will need to be fused and monitored in real time. Multimodality imaging and sensing of biologic and physiologic data likely will be important. As is becoming increasingly true for diagnostic imaging, quantitative imaging will likely be important during IGI necessitating rigorous standardization of the imaging used for real-time guidance, monitoring, and endpoint determination as well as longer-term imaging follow-up (see QIBA for more details; https://www.rsna.org/QIBA.aspx). Endpoint determination and continued postprocedural surveillance using such methods will also likely be of importance and become used with increased frequency. Therefore the development and validation of these imaging methods will be critical. These will require clinical trials of various designs. Similarly, combination therapies are already becoming more prevalent. The integration between these therapies and the integration of the local–regional therapies with the imaging guidance will need to become "tighter." These integrations will also require development and validation through clinical trials. Horizontal translation of IGIs from one intended clinical utility to another and from one clinical condition to another will need to become more facile and economical while still developing the requisite data to support evidence-based decision-making. This will require advances in clinical trial design and conduct.

The realization of these futures will require the active collaboration among IGI physician–scientists, biostatisticians, ethicists, federal agencies, and industry sponsors. A firm understanding of the design, implementation, and conduct of IGI clinical trials must be the foundation upon which this collaboration takes place.

References

1 Dhruva, S.S., L.A. Bero, and R.F. Redberg, Strength of study evidence examined by the FDA in premarket approval of cardiovascular devices. *JAMA*, 2009. **302**(24): p. 2679–2685.

2 Challoner, D., et al., *Medical Devices and the Public's Health: The FDA 510(k) Clearance Process at 35 Years.* 2011, The National Academies Press: Washington, DC. p. 280.

3 Colevas, A.D., et al., Development of investigational radiation modifiers. *J Natl Cancer Inst*, 2003. **95**(9): p. 646–651.

4 Liu, F.-F., et al., Lessons learned from radiation oncology clinical trials. *Clin Cancer Res*, 2013. **19**(22): p. 6089–6100.

5 Spigel, D.R., et al., Tracheoesophageal fistula formation in patients with lung cancer treated with chemoradiation and bevacizumab. *J Clin Oncol*, 2010. **28**(1): p. 43–48.

6 Hahn, S.M., et al., A Phase I trial of the farnesyltransferase inhibitor L-778,123 and radiotherapy for locally advanced lung and head and neck cancer. *Clin Cancer Res*, 2002. **8**(5): p. 1065–1072.

7 Martin, N.E., et al., A phase I trial of the dual farnesyltransferase and geranylgeranyltransferase inhibitor L-778,123 and radiotherapy for locally advanced pancreatic cancer. *Clin Cancer Res*, 2004. **10**(16): p. 5447–5454.

8 Rengan, R., et al., A phase I trial of the HIV protease inhibitor nelfinavir with concurrent chemoradiotherapy for unresectable stage IIIA/IIIB non-small cell lung cancer: a report of toxicities and clinical response. *J Thorac Oncol*, 2012. **7**(4): p. 709–715.

9 Willett, C.G., et al., A safety and survival analysis of neoadjuvant bevacizumab with standard chemoradiation in a phase I/II study compared with standard chemoradiation in locally advanced rectal cancer. *Oncologist*, 2010. **15**(8): p. 845–851.

10 Harrington, K.J., et al., Two-stage phase I dose-escalation study of intratumoral reovirus type 3 dearing and palliative radiotherapy in patients with advanced cancers. *Clin Cancer Res*, 2010. **16**(11): p. 3067–3077.

11 Willett, C.G., et al., Complete pathological response to bevacizumab and chemoradiation in advanced rectal cancer. *Nat Clin Pract Oncol*, 2007. **4**(5): p. 316–321.

12 Willett, C.G., et al., Direct evidence that the VEGF-specific antibody bevacizumab has antivascular effects in human rectal cancer. *Nat Med*, 2004. **10**(2): p. 145–147.

13 Ben-Josef, E., et al., A phase I/II trial of intensity modulated radiation (IMRT) dose escalation with concurrent fixed-dose rate gemcitabine (FDR-G) in patients with unresectable pancreatic cancer. *Int J Radiat Oncol Biol Phys*, 2012. **84**(5): p. 1166–1171.

14 Pijls-Johannesma, M., et al., A systematic methodology review of phase I radiation dose escalation trials. *Radiother Oncol*, 2010. **95**(2): p. 135–141.

15 Eisenhauer, E.A., et al., New response evaluation criteria in solid tumours: revised RECIST guideline (version 1.1). *Eur J Cancer*, 2009. **45**(2): p. 228–247.

16 Wahl, R.L., et al., From RECIST to PERCIST: evolving considerations for PET response criteria in solid tumors. *J Nucl Med*, 2009. **50**(Suppl 1): p. 122s–150s.

17 Bruix, J., et al., Clinical management of hepatocellular carcinoma. Conclusions of the Barcelona-2000 EASL conference. European Association for the Study of the Liver. *J Hepatol*, 2001. **35**(3): p. 421–430.

18 Lencioni, R. and J.M. Llovet, Modified RECIST (mRECIST) assessment for hepatocellular carcinoma. *Semin Liver Dis*, 2010. **30**(1): p. 52–60.

19 Hurwitz, M.D., et al., Magnetic resonance-guided focused ultrasound for patients with painful bone metastases: phase III trial results. *J Natl Cancer Inst*, 2014. **106**(5).

20 Smith, G.C. and J.P. Pell, Parachute use to prevent death and major trauma related to gravitational challenge: systematic review of randomised controlled trials. *BMJ*, 2003. **327**(7429): p. 1459–1461.

CHAPTER 4

Imaging as a predictor of therapeutic response

David A. Mankoff[1] and Anthony F. Shields[2]

[1] *University of Pennsylvania, Philadelphia, PA, USA*
[2] *Barbara Ann Karmanos Cancer Institute, Wayne State University, Detroit, MI, USA*

KEY POINTS

- In addition to their role in diagnosis, imaging tests are valuable as biomarkers to guide patient treatment.
- Imaging-based and tissue-based biomarkers are complementary.
- The categories of imaging biomarkers include prognostic markers, predictive markers, early response indicators, and predictors of therapeutic outcome or surrogate endpoints.
- Ultimately, all biomarker applications have the goal of predicting and improving key patient outcomes such as progression-free or overall survival and may serve as surrogate endpoints for clinical trials in settings where they are sufficiently predictive of survival.
- Before a biomarker can be applied to clinical trials and clinical practice, its analytic validity must be tested and proven in early studies, including the establishment of standard methods, assessment of reproducibility, and comparison against a reference standard.

4.1 Introduction

In this chapter, we review the applications of imaging as a predictor of therapeutic outcome, that is, as a disease biomarker. We define biomarker in the context of disease treatment and review the types of biomarkers used to direct therapy. We emphasize cancer applications, where both tissue and imaging biomarkers have been widely studied [1]; however, the concepts provided are equally applicable to other diseases.

Handbook for Clinical Trials of Imaging and Image-Guided Interventions, First Edition.
Edited by Nancy A. Obuchowski and G. Scott Gazelle.

4.1.1 What is a biomarker?

The term **biomarker** is used to describe a biologic measure that characterizes disease status and/or predicts disease behavior [1]. With the goal of increasingly individualized treatment, biomarkers have become an increasingly important part of clinical care [1]. Biomarkers can be used to detect disease; for example, PSA is used for prostate cancer screening. Biomarkers can also be used to direct therapy, which is the focus of this chapter.

4.1.2 Why do we need imaging biomarkers to direct therapy?

The ability to assay biologic features of disease and the impact of therapy on the disease biology are fundamental to the development of new treatments, their testing in clinical trials, and their use in clinical practice [2]. Advances in our ability to measure genomics, gene expression, protein expression, and cellular biology have led to a host of new targets for drug therapy. In translating new drugs into clinical trials and clinical practice, these same methods serve to identify subjects most likely to benefit from specific treatments. As medicine and therapeutic decision-making become more individualized and targeted, there is an increasing need to characterize diseases and identify therapeutic targets, in order to select therapy most likely to be successful. An example is the identification of HER2 overexpression to predict response to HER2-directed therapies such as trastuzumab and lapatinib [3]. There is a complementary need to assay cancer drug pharmacodynamics, namely, the effect of a particular drug on the disease, to determine whether or not the drug has "hit" the target and whether the drug is likely to be effective in curing the disease, for example, by eliminating the cancer from a patient [4]. This is particularly important in early drug trials as proof of mechanism and prediction of the likelihood of disease activity in patients.

Thus far most assays used to identify therapeutic targets or drug pharmacodynamics have been based upon *in vitro* assays of tissue material or blood samples. Advances in both technology and cancer science have led to the ability to perform noninvasive molecular assays. An example is the use of reporter genes, generally used in rodents, whose expression results in the production of material such as green fluorescent protein or luciferase that can be detected without tissue sampling [5]. Another advance, applicable to the entire range of biological systems from cell culture to humans, is imaging biomarkers, both anatomically based measures such as CT, and more recently functional and molecularly based methods such as PET [6, 7]. Imaging as a marker for therapeutic outcome can be considered an *in vivo* assay technique capable of measuring regional tumor biology and the impact of therapy without perturbing either [8, 9].

4.1.3 Types of therapeutic biomarkers

Biomarkers for therapeutic trials are often divided into four types: (i) prognostic, (ii) predictive, (iii) early response, and (iv) predictors of therapeutic outcome. These are described later, listed in Table 4.1, and illustrated in Figure 4.1.

Table 4.1 Type of predictive biomarkers.

Prognostic
- Indicates disease aggressiveness and the likelihood of death and/or disease progression
- Independent of treatment

Predictive
- Predicts the likelihood of therapeutic benefit from a specific treatment
- Often linked to therapeutic targets or resistance factors

Early response
- Provides an early indicator of therapeutic response as a predictor of later therapeutic benefits
- Often measures drug pharmacodynamics, that is, measures of drug action on the disease

Therapeutic benefit
- A marker of therapeutic benefit that predicts key outcomes such as overall survival, progression-free survival, etc.
- With sufficient validation, can be considered a surrogate endpoint for therapeutic trials

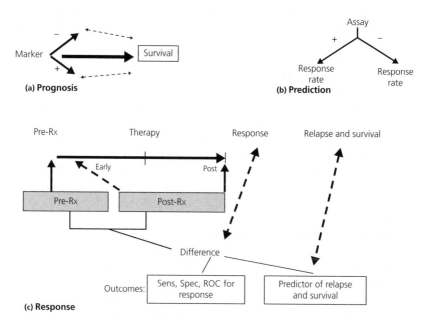

Figure 4.1 Illustrations for different types of therapeutic markers. Diagrams illustrate trials for (a) prognostic, (b) predictive, and (c) response (early response and therapeutic benefit) markers. The response marker illustration shows a timeline for response and indicates trial designs for testing early response indicators ("early" label in the timeline) as well as predictors of therapeutic benefit that can serve as surrogate endpoints for longer-term outcomes such as relapse and survival.

Prognostic markers are a class of predictive markers that assess the aggressiveness of an individual patient's disease and the likelihood it will lead to death. The most common use for prognostic markers is in the prediction of death from disease or in some cases the likelihood of disease progression or relapse (see Chapter 10 for a statistical description of these outcomes). In principle, prognostic measures are intrinsic to the patient and the disease and are independent of treatment. In practice, however, it can be difficult to separate the effect of the disease and the therapeutic intervention in the exploration of a particular biomarker as a prognostic marker.

Predictive markers describe the likelihood of a patient's response to a specific therapy for a particular disease. Predictive markers depend upon both disease features and the choice of treatment. The goal for predictive markers can be objective response, disease-free survival (DFS) or progression-free survival (PFS), or overall survival (OS) (see Chapter 10). In practice, markers may have both prognostic and predictive features. An example is estrogen receptor (ER) expression in breast cancer. ER expression is both a prognostic and predictive marker. ER expression predicts a less aggressive tumor and more favorable disease course compared to ER nonexpressing tumors. In addition, a lack of ER expression predicts that breast cancer response to endocrine therapy is unlikely [10]. More recent examples include multigene assays for cancer such as Oncotype DX for breast cancer, which has helped predict tumor behavior and therapeutic response and is used to determine the need for aggressive treatment such as adjuvant chemotherapy [11].

Early response markers indicate whether or not there has been evidence of response to treatment, namely, that the chosen therapy has hit its therapeutic target and produced an effect on the disease. These are also called pharmacodynamic markers in that they indicate a cellular response to drug therapy. Pharmacodynamic markers provide an early indication that the chosen therapy may work. Equally if not more importantly, these markers can identify a lack of response and therefore predict therapeutic futility. An example of a tissue-based early response indicator is serial assay of tumor proliferation for cancer, for example, using Ki-67 immunohistochemistry, to assess early response to breast cancer endocrine therapy [12].

Predictors of therapeutic outcome, often called a surrogate endpoint, is a marker of therapeutic success that is strongly associated with long-term patient outcomes such as DFS, PFS, or OS (see Chapter 10). An example of a tissue surrogate endpoint is complete pathologic response of breast cancer to presurgical (neoadjuvant) systemic therapy, which has been accepted by the US Food and Drug Administration (FDA) as a surrogate endpoint for efficacy of breast cancer treatment based upon its ability to predict DFS [13]. In some cases, DFS measured at a specific time point can serve as a marker for OS. For example, 3-year DFS in patients receiving adjuvant treatment for stage II–III colon cancer now regularly serves as a marker for OS, which can require five or more years to accurately measure.

4.2 Imaging- versus tissue-based biomarkers

It is important to keep in perspective inherent differences in capabilities between tissue-based assays and *in vivo* assays using imaging. Imaging is noninvasive and therefore better suited to serial assay. This is especially important in imaging specific drug pharmacodynamics and early response. In addition, imaging typically surveys the entire animal or patient and therefore avoids sampling error that can occur for assays that require tissue sampling, especially when there is significant disease heterogeneity. However, while sample-based methods can assay many different processes at once, for example, the expression of an array of genes [14], imaging can typically sample one or at most a few processes at the same time. Also, while it is possible to "batch" processing for many samples at the same time, imaging needs to be performed one subject at a time. Furthermore, the need for sophisticated equipment and imaging probes makes imaging typically more expensive than sample-based assay. These last two factors limit the number of subjects that can be studied by imaging compared to sample assay. In general, imaging methods are complementary to assay-based methods and best used to test novel drugs in the late stages of preclinical testing and early clinical trials, with more focused and limited use of imaging in later-stage drug trials.

4.3 Examples of imaging biomarker applications

4.3.1 Prognostic markers

Prognostic markers indicate disease aggressiveness and the likelihood that the disease will cause the patient significant harm, including the chance that the disease will lead to the patient's death. In practice, prognostic markers are important in matching the aggressiveness (and accompanying side effects) of treatment to the severity of the disease. Examples for cancer include measures of cellular proliferation, such as the Ki-67, which indicates the expected rate of disease progression in the absence of therapy and therefore predicts the need for more aggressive treatment in a number of cancers [15].

There are a number of examples of imaging as a prognostic marker. The level of FDG uptake in many cancers at the time of diagnosis or recurrence has been shown to be predictive of downstream outcomes such as OS, DFS, and PFS [7, 9]. An important example commonly used in clinical practice relates treatment for patients with recurrent and/or metastatic thyroid cancer who fail to respond to $^{131}I^-$. In such cases, alternative therapies often carry significant toxicities and may not be required for more indolent disease. In this setting, the absence of thyroid cancer FDG uptake, as assessed by FDG PET/CT, has been shown to be predictive of an indolent tumor and prolonged survival (Figure 4.2). In a landmark study, Wang and colleagues [17] showed in a retrospective analysis that patients with iodine-refractory thyroid cancer that was FDG negative were highly unlikely to die of their disease, while patients whose tumors with FDG uptake had 50%

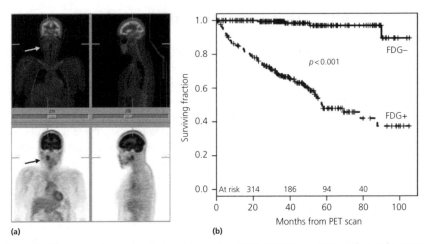

(a)   (b)

Figure 4.2 Example of a prognostic imaging marker. FDG PET/CT can detect iodine-refractory thyroid cancer recurrence and/or metastasis **(a)**, in this case in an unusual location (parapharyngeal space). The presence of FDG uptake in iodine-refractory thyroid cancer has been shown to be extraordinarily prognostic **(b)** [16] in that patients whose tumors do not take up FDG are very unlikely to die of their disease.

mortality in less than 5 years, indicating an aggressive variant of thyroid cancer warranting further treatment. The key prognostic information provided by FDG PET in this setting is commonly used in clinical decision-making for iodine-refractory thyroid cancer and has been used to select patients for trials of novel thyroid cancer therapy [18].

Another example of a prognostic marker uniquely indicated by imaging studies is tumor hypoxia, which has been shown to result in a more aggressive phenotype, more likely to lead to clinical aggressive tumor behavior and death [19]. Hypoxia is difficult to gauge by tissue sampling; however, several imaging approaches can provide quantitative estimates of the extent and severity of tumor hypoxia, including PET with hypoxia imaging agents such as ^{18}F-fluoromisonidazole (FMISO) and ^{60}Cu-ATSM, as well as BOLD MRI and other MR-based methods. PET hypoxia imaging in brain tumors, head and neck cancer, and cervical cancer have all shown the prognostic value of hypoxia imaging, predicting important outcomes such as OS and PFS in patients with these cancer types [16, 20, 21]. These trials had a common design testing the hypoxia imaging agent as an integrated (i.e., observational only) biomarker in a population of patients with a common disease at a specific time point (either at diagnosis or recurrence prior to therapy) and comparing tracer uptake to PFS or OS. For example, in the study of FMISO PET by Spence et al. [21], patients were imaged prior to radiotherapy and followed for tumor progression and/or death. Previously established measures of hypoxia based on FMISO uptake (hypoxic volume and maximum tumor/blood ratio) were included in single-variable and multivariable Cox proportional hazards models (see Chapter 10 for a description of this method) for time to progression and survival and showed significant predictive value that was independent of other established markers such as tumor volume. These early results spurred later multicenter trials in the same clinical setting.

4.3.2 Predictive markers

Predictive markers play a key role in directing therapy, especially as treatment becomes more individualized and directed at specific therapeutic targets [22]. In clinical practice, predictive assays, often measures of therapeutic target expression, are commonly used to select treatment. In many cases, the most important finding may be the absence of an expected therapeutic target, which would direct the patient toward alternative therapy. One of the most established markers in cancer is the ER, which is widely used to direct endocrine therapy in breast cancer [10]. In breast cancers expressing ER, the chance of therapeutic response to endocrine therapy is as high as 75%, but in the absence of expression, therapeutic benefit occurs in less than 5% of patients. Thus in clinical practice, a negative ER assay (i.e., showing no evidence of ER expression) has a direct effect on patient management [10]. PET imaging of ER expression using the positron-emitting probe, ^{18}F-fluoroestradiol (FES), has been tested as a predictive measure for breast cancer endocrine therapy, with good initial success [23, 24] (Figure 4.3). In these trials, FES PET was performed as a purely observational marker in patients with locally advanced or metastatic breast cancer prior to undergoing treatment with endocrine therapy (targeted to the ER), spurred by prior studies showing that the level of FES uptake correlated with the presence of ER expression in the tumor, assessed by *in vitro* assays of biopsy material. The level of FES uptake was compared for patients who subsequently had a response by standard clinical assessment criteria compared to those not responding to endocrine therapy. These studies found a higher average FES SUV for responders versus nonresponders, and both indicated a mean FES SUV across disease sites of 1.5 as a threshold below which patients were unlikely to respond to endocrine treatment. In addition to providing a noninvasive predictive assay for endocrine therapy, the ability to characterize ER expression over the entire disease burden may offer advantages for patients with more widespread disease, especially when the disease has spread to locations where biopsy is difficult, such as bone. This advantage, combined with promising early results in single-center trials, has led to the development of multicenter trials to further establish FES PET as a predictive assay for breast cancer endocrine therapy.

Another example of imaging to direct target treatment is hypoxia imaging. One application lies in radiotherapy, where hypoxia has shown to be resistance to photon treatment [19]. In this case, hypoxia imaging can be used to identify hypoxic tumor regions that will require higher doses of radiation, information that can be incorporated into radiotherapy treatment plans [25]. Hypoxia imaging is also a key predictive assay for hypoxic radiosensitizers and hypoxia-selective chemotherapeutic agents. A key example can be found in the study of Rischin and colleagues [26], in a trial of the hypoxia-selective cancer agent, tirapazamine, in

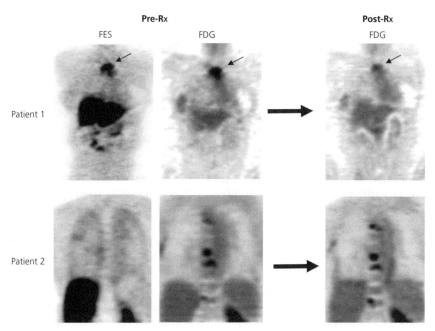

Figure 4.3 Example of a predictive imaging biomarker. Images illustrate the correlation between ^{18}F-fluoroestradiol (FES) uptake, as a measure of breast cancer ER expression and as predictive assay for and subsequent response to hormonal therapy. Coronal images of FES uptake (left column) and FDG (middle column) uptake pretherapy, along with FDG uptake posthormonal therapy (right column), are shown for two patients (top and bottom row). The patient in the top row had a sternal recurrence of breast cancer that had high FES uptake (arrow; image also shows liver and bowel uptake, both normal findings). FDG images taken before and after 6 weeks of letrozole treatment show a significant decline in FDG uptake, with subsequent excellent clinical response. The patient in the bottom row had newly diagnosed metastatic breast cancer with an ER+ primary tumor by immunohistochemistry. However, there was no FES uptake at multiple bone metastases seen by FDG PET. The patient failed endocrine therapy, as indicated by the lack of change in the posttherapy FDG PET. The level of FES uptake, as an indicator of therapeutic target (ER) expression, was predictive of the likelihood of therapeutic response.

advanced head and neck cancer, a cancer that is often hypoxic. In this trial, patients with advanced head and neck cancer were randomized to receive radiotherapy and standard chemotherapy versus radiotherapy and a tirapazamine-containing chemotherapy regimen. In the overall population, tirapazamine failed to demonstrate a therapeutic benefit, and the overall trial (and drug) failed. However, in the subset of patients who underwent an exploratory FMISO PET scan prior to treatment (an **integrated marker**, not used to direct therapy), patients with evidence of hypoxia by FMISO PET showed significantly better response and PFS when treated with tirapazamine compared to standard chemotherapy. Had FMISO PET been used to select patients for the trial, it is likely that the trial would have shown benefit for tirapazamine. This example serves to indicate the significant role that image-based biomarkers can play in patient selection for clinical trials and clinical practice. Trials using such an **integral marker** utilize the biomarker to help select patients for a given therapy (see Section 4.4.2 for further details about integrated and integral markers).

4.3.3 Early response markers

The standard clinical approach to the assessment of response in patients undergoing chemotherapy or radiation for advanced disease is measurement of the size of the tumor about every 2 months (usual range: 6 weeks to 3 months) using standard anatomic imaging with CT or MRI. This is meant to allow enough time for a tumor to shrink in responding patients or to grow in those with progressive disease. The exact timing depends on the tumor being treated, the likely response to treatment, and the availability of other treatment options. While similar assessments are usually employed for patients receiving routine treatment as well as those enrolled on clinical trials, at times research trials require more frequent assessments, especially when PFS is the primary outcome of a study. It should be kept in mind that assessment that falls within the standard of care can usually be justified and paid for by insurance, while more frequent assessments may require funding as part of the study.

The limitations of standard anatomic imaging, such as those using RECIST 1.1, need to be kept in mind when being performed to monitor therapy. A slow-growing tumor may not change in size over a couple of months, but be perfectly viable and grow over a longer period of time. This can be evident in studies comparing a new agent to a placebo, where it still may take some time for progression to become evident. For example, in a trial of everolimus in advanced pancreatic neuroendocrine tumor, those on the placebo arm had a median PFS of 4.6 months [27]. While results in the placebo arm were clearly worse than the treated arm (PFS 11.0 months, $p < 0.001$), many patients did not rapidly progress and 9% on the placebo arm were progression-free at 19 months. On the other hand, in responding patients the tumor may take some time for the lesion to become necrotic and actually shrink in size. This has become an issue with some of the new, targeted agents that may lead to tumor necrosis without an appreciable change in size or even some enlargement. For example, early in the course of treatment, in patients with gastrointestinal stromal tumors, imatinib may lead to an increase in tumor size but a decrease in tumor density or even the appearance of new low-density lesions in the liver, which were not previously visible [28]. New imaging criteria are being developed for such situations. The recent successes in immunotherapy of cancer have further clouded the picture when using anatomic imaging. The inflammatory response generated from such treatments, such as seen with the antibody ipilimumab against cytotoxic T-lymphocyte antigen-4 (CTLA-4) or nivolumab the anti-PD-1 antibody, can also lead to increases in the size of tumors or the appearances of new, previously unseen lesions [29]. This has led to protocols using such agents to allow investigators to continue treatment

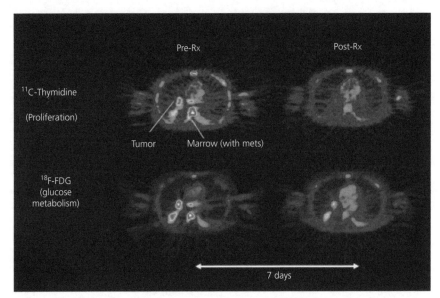

Figure 4.4 Example of proliferation imaging an early response indicator. PET images of
[11]C-thymidine (top) and FDG (bottom) uptake pre- and 7 days postchemotherapy in a patient
with small-cell lung cancer undergoing chemotherapy are shown. Both measures show a
decline in uptake early after treatment in a patient that went on to have a complete clinical
response for 1 year. The dramatic response seen in the thymidine images is an illustration of
the potential utility of PET proliferation as an early response indicator. Source: Shields [31].
Reproduced with permission from Society of Nuclear Medicine and Molecular Imaging.

when early in therapy tumors are found to shrink, remain stable, or even increase
in size. Clearly, new approaches are needed in these situations.

Functional and molecular imaging methods may be able to identify change in
response to treatment earlier than size-based methods and have been studied and
tested as early response indicators. One method particularly well suited to this task
is PET proliferation imaging [30]. A decline in proliferation provides an early indicator of therapeutic success that works for both cytotoxic and cytostatic therapies.
Much of this work so far has focused on labeled thymidine and thymidine analogs
used for PET. Early studies with ^{11}C-thymidine demonstrated the ability of this
approach to measure response soon after therapy administration (Figure 4.4) [31].
More recently, the thymidine analog ^{18}F-fluorothymidine (FLT) has been tested as
an indicator of early response, with success for several treatment and cancer types
[32, 33]. In the study by Kenny et al. [32], FLT imaging was performed as an observational marker pretherapy and after a single round of epirubicin-based chemotherapy in patients with advanced breast cancer. Pretherapy FLT PET was repeated
in a subset of patients to measure the test/retest reproducibility (see Chapter 10 for
a description of this study design) for FLT uptake measures. The fractional change
in FLT uptake pre- and 1 week posttherapy was compared to subsequent lesion-
based clinical response using size criteria. Responding lesions showed an average

decline in FLT uptake of 41% compared to a 3% increase in uptake for nonresponding lesions and a mean test/retest difference of 11%. These results formed the basis for a later multicenter trial in the same clinical setting, which confirmed the value of FLT PET as an early response indicator [34].

4.3.4 Therapeutic benefit markers and surrogate measurements for long-term outcomes

Ultimately, the outcome desired for any cancer therapy is to improve survival in patients with advanced disease. OS still serves as the primary outcome in patients with particularly poor prognoses and relatively short median survival times. For example, a recent trial in advanced pancreatic cancer has demonstrated the median survival improved to 8.5 months from 6.7 months when nab-paclitaxel was added to the standard regimen of single agent gemcitabine [35]. Obviously, survival is the most clear-cut endpoint, but it is difficult to assess the role of a single therapy when patients have multiple treatment options available and generally receive a series of agents over the course of time that can stretch into many years. Fortunately, from the patient's perspective, this clinical situation is now regularly encountered in the treatment of breast, colon, and prostate cancers where prolonged survival in those with advanced disease is now the norm. Hence, imaging endpoints are commonly used as a surrogate marker and have generally supplanted survival as the primary endpoint, except in those with refractory disease. Response rate, the fraction of patients with tumor shrinkage, has generally been replaced with the assessment of PFS as the primary objective in many such trials. Many of the successful, newer targeted agents can greatly improve time to progression while having minimal impact on response. For example, a randomized trial of sunitinib versus placebo in patients with GIST refractory to imatinib demonstrated that the PFS was 27.3 and 6.4 weeks, respectively ($p<0.001$) [36]. On the other hand, sunitinib only had a response rate of 7%. This trial allowed for crossover in patients progressing on placebo, which can blunt any survival differences, although in this study survival was improved on the arm receiving sunitinib first.

An illustrative example of an early study to test a putative imaging-based therapeutic benefit marker is shown in Figure 4.5. ^{99m}Tc-sestamibi (MIBI) is a SPECT tracer used for myocardial perfusion and for cancer detection, and it showed effectiveness in measuring therapeutic response in women undergoing neoadjuvant therapy for breast cancer [37, 39]. Early studies showed that a semiquantitative index of MIBI uptake was able to classify patients by whether or not they achieved a complete pathologic response (pCR), a well-established surrogate endpoint for neoadjuvant chemotherapy [40]. In these studies, MIBI imaging was performed as an integrated (observational) marker pretherapy, midtherapy, and posttherapy in patients with locally advanced breast cancer undergoing neoadjuvant (presurgical) chemotherapy and compared to pathologic response to therapy assessed at posttherapy surgery. Based upon prior analysis showing an acceptable interobserver (18%) and intraobserver (11%) variability, the ratio of tumor to normal breast uptake was chosen as a quantitative marker for these

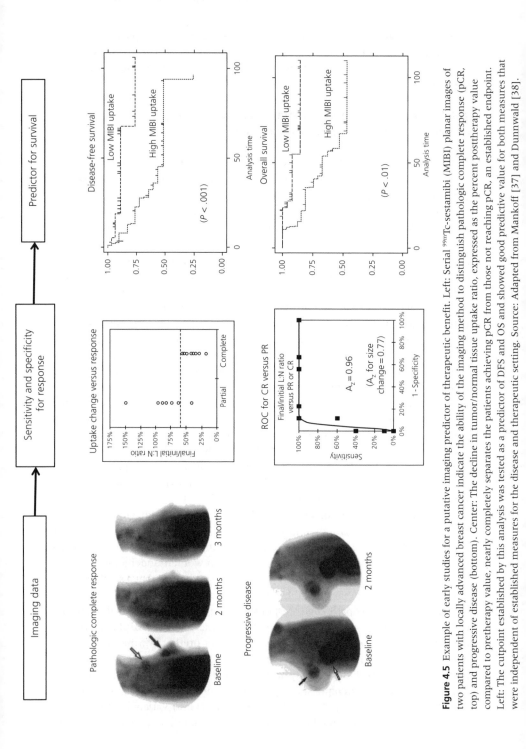

Figure 4.5 Example of early studies for a putative imaging predictor of therapeutic benefit. Left: Serial ^{99m}Tc-sestamibi (MIBI) planar images of two patients with locally advanced breast cancer indicate the ability of the imaging method to distinguish pathologic complete response (pCR, top) and progressive disease (bottom). Center: The decline in tumor/normal tissue uptake ratio, expressed as the percent posttherapy value compared to pretherapy value, nearly completely separates the patients achieving pCR from those not reaching pCR, an established endpoint. Left: The cutpoint established by this analysis was tested as a predictor of DFS and OS and showed good predictive value for both measures that were independent of established measures for the disease and therapeutic setting. Source: Adapted from Mankoff [37] and Dunnwald [38].

studies. The MIBI uptake indices declined a mean of 58% in patients achieving a pCR compared to a mean decline of 18% in patients with a clinical response but residual tumor posttherapy (partial response, not pCR). ROC analysis showed area under the curve $(A_z) > 0.9$ for classifying response as pCR versus not pCR and established cutoffs for the change in MIBI uptake as a predictor of pCR [38] (see Chapter 9 for a discussion on ROC analysis). Subsequent studies with additional patients and clinical follow-up showed that the change in MIBI uptake predicted key therapeutic outcomes (DFS, OS), providing prognostic information independent of and incremental to established predictors, including pCR [41] (see Chapter 8 for a discussion of statistical modeling). This example provides an illustration of the early steps in testing a therapeutic benefit marker, which would now require larger, multicenter trials to gain more widespread application.

4.4 Approach to biomarker study design

4.4.1 Standards for biomarker clinical trial design and results reporting

Consensus definitions of the essential features for biomarker research have been defined in guidelines for the validation and use of biomarkers in clinical trials and clinical care. This has been most widely accepted for cancer clinical trials [1, 42]. The REMARK guidelines are the most widely accepted reporting criteria for cancer biomarker trials [42]. Important features of these guidelines and biomarker trial reporting include the following [1, 42]: determination of the analytic validity of the biomarker, including calibration, precision, and accuracy of the measurement; the intended use for directing cancer therapy; the magnitude of the biomarker's clinical value; and the quality of the clinical trial data supporting the biomarker. The analytic validity of the marker describes the existence of an accepted and tested method to perform the measurement, the threshold for considering the biomarker positive or negative (if applicable), and the reproducibility of the measurement (see Chapter 10). The magnitude of the biomarker's predictive value and the quality of clinical trial data supporting biomarker use are key factors in the clinical acceptance of the biomarker (see Chapter 10). The strongest level of evidence (level 1) supporting a biomarker comes from prospective clinical trials specifically designed to test the impact of the biomarker on patient outcome [1, 41, 42] (see Chapter 11). This requires studies designed to compare patient treatments and outcome when the biomarker is used (integral marker) to the case where the disease is treated without input from the biomarker. This type of design can be challenging for imaging biomarkers, where clinical trials can be expensive and may not provide benefit for the patient. An alternative approach is to test the biomarker in a purely observational study with prospectively defined biomarker endpoints considered level 2 evidence [41, 42]. For example, studies leading to the FDA approval of multigene assays for breast cancer came from studies where the results of the assay were applied in a retrospective (observational only) fashion to data from randomized controlled adjuvant therapy trials to validate their value in predicting the need for chemotherapy to prevent recurrence [11]. In practice, some biomarkers are used with lesser levels of evidence, but may not be approved as diagnostic markers, since this typically requires level 1 or good level 2 evidence.

4.4.2 Integral versus integrated biomarkers

There are a number of different approaches to biomarker validation: the biomarker may be tested in a purely observational fashion or may be used to direct therapy as part of an experimental study [22]. The terms "integral" and "integrated" are used to describe the different types of biomarker use in a clinical trial [42, 43]. An **integral biomarker** directly affects the clinical trial and is essential to trial conduct. Integral biomarkers affect the patient path through clinical trial procedures, for example, to direct stratification between arms of a treatment study. Integral biomarkers are typically biomarkers where the analytic method has been extensively validated in prior trials. Study design that includes an integral biomarker can provide level 1 evidence supporting the biomarker for the specific indication tested in the trial. For example, interim FDG PET/CT early in the course of lymphoma treatment can be used as an integral biomarker to direct subsequent treatment, a common feature in recent lymphoma therapy trials [44]. In cases where clinical trials with an integral biomarker prove that a particular drug or drug combination is effective, the biomarker can become part of the drug indication for use in clinical practice and is required for the use of that particular drug.

Integrated biomarkers are markers that are measured in the context of a prospective trial but are not used to direct treatment. Once validated as an integrated biomarker, biomarkers may be used as integral biomarkers in subsequent clinical trials using information from the integrated biomarker trials to set thresholds for directing trial procedures, such as choice of treatment [22]. As an example of integrated biomarker study design and the approach to developing markers suitable for serving as integrated markers, we return to Case example 1.2 in Chapter 1, testing FDG PET as an early indicator of response to biologically directed therapy in breast cancer. In this case, the biologic target is the HER2 molecule. When overexpressed, the HER2 offers a potential target for therapy directed against HER2, such as trastuzumab. However, not all patients respond to HER2-targeted therapy, and HER2-targeted therapy is frequently used in combination with chemotherapy, making the contribution of the targeted therapy to tumor response difficult to discern. These factors motivate the need for an early response indicator for HER2-directed therapy. Early single-center studies testing FDG PET in small trials of patients undergoing HER2-directed therapy compared the change in FDG uptake to subsequent response and suggested that FDG PET might be an early indicator of response to HER2-targeted therapy. The utility of FDG PET/CT was directly tested in the NeoALTTO trial, where three different combinations of HER2-directed therapy, given in combination with paclitaxel, were compared using pathologic response as the endpoint. The trial design included a "biologic window" where the HER2-targeted agents were used without paclitaxel, providing the ideal setting for testing FDG PET/CT as an early response indicator for HER2-directed therapy in the setting of a well-controlled therapy trial [45]. Serial FDG PET/CT scans were obtained in this trial with the goal of testing FDG PET/CT as an early marker of HER2-directed drug efficacy. The study showed a significant difference in FDG decline with HER2-directed therapy for patients achieving pCR versus those that did not and indicated the capability of FDG PET/CT to discriminate responders from nonresponders. However, the data did not indicate an optimal threshold for predicting a lack of good response (no pCR), indicating a possible limitation to using serial FDG PET/CT as an integral marker to choose patients for HER2-directed therapy in subsequent trials. This prompted a call for further studies of FDG PET/CT in this setting and possibly alternative approaches.

4.4.3 Altering therapy with early response markers

Assessment of response soon after the start of treatment may be used to discontinue treatment that is predicted, with a high degree of certainty, to fail to benefit the patient. For a biomarker to find utility in such a situation requires rigorous testing and a full understanding of the timing of the assessment, its predictive value, and utility of alternate treatments. For example, an FDG PET obtained in esophageal adenocarcinoma patients about two weeks after the start of neoadjuvant chemotherapy was able to demonstrate which patients were not likely to respond to treatment, when tested as an integrated marker [46]. A subsequent phase II trial used this early treatment biomarker to select responding patients to continue treatment with the chemotherapy, while nonresponding patients were switched to radiotherapy [47]. In this trial, patients with advanced adenocarcinoma of the gastroesophageal junction underwent FDG PET pretherapy and after 14 days of chemotherapy. Patients were classified as PET response versus nonresponders on the basis of thresholds for the decline in FDG uptake established in prior studies. PET responders continued treatment with chemotherapy, whereas PET nonresponders switched to chemoradiotherapy, a more toxic but potentially more effective regimen. Unfortunately, patients not responding to chemotherapy, based on the scans, did equally poorly when chemoradiotherapy was used. Hence, imaging in this situation provided a strong prognostic marker, but did little to improve outcome, in large part due to the lack of an effective therapy for metabolic nonresponders. While the use of FDG PET as an early biomarker for esophageal cancer may lead to insights in subsequent trials and improvements using new treatment approaches, at present it cannot be recommended for use as an early response indicator for routine therapy of esophageal carcinoma. This is unlike the situation in lymphoma where alternate successful treatment approaches are available, as noted previously, and an early therapy, "interim" PET scan is used in many clinical practices. Hence, the utility of an early biomarker in changing therapy will depend not only on the accuracy of the marker but also in the availability of alternate, potentially successful treatment approaches to improve the patient outcome. This may be a rapidly changing arena as both new biomarkers and treatments become available. Furthermore, a biomarker that works with a given disease and treatment may not work when being used with a different disease or modality.

4.5 Practical considerations

The previous discussion has highlighted some of the main issues that must be taken into account when developing biomarkers to predict treatment response and the need to validate these approaches in the context of the changing availability and knowledge about the accuracy of various markers and their application to results with standard and new treatments. Furthermore, it must be kept in mind that optimal use of the biomarker may depend on the timing relative to the start of treatment. One major issue is the cost and difficulty in obtaining, validating, and using biomarkers. For tissue biomarkers, this may include the cost of repeated biopsies and tumor analysis, which can be considerable. These costs may exceed those of sophisticated imaging with novel PET or MR approaches. Over the last decade, the cost of treatment has skyrocketed. As a result, biomarkers may be very cost-effective if they can help select patients who will or are benefiting from treatment. In general, such biomarkers are more commonly used to determine which patients are not likely to benefit from treatment. For example, the cost of the anti-EGFR antibody cetuximab, for the treatment of advanced colorectal cancer, is about $5000 per month. It has been found that patients with KRAS mutations do not benefit from such therapy, and in addition to the cost of treatment, they may experience significant toxicity, while other treatment options are withheld [48]. Even with such testing, further early measures of response or failure are being sought, since only a minority of patients appear to respond to therapy. Further refinements seek to find additional subgroups of patients who are unlikely to benefit from such therapy, including those with NRAS and BRAF mutations, as well as those who do not overexpress the EGFR ligands. The development of new biomarkers, both tissue and imaging, is also being vigorously pursued for the assessment of antivascular agents. A number of such agents, both antibodies and small molecules, are available and used in the treatment of a number of tumor types, but we lack any reliable biomarkers tied to outcome. This has led to the unusual situation where bevacizumab was initially approved by the FDA for the treatment of breast cancer based on measurement of PFS, but approval was subsequently withdrawn when survival was found to be unchanged. This highlights the need for biomarkers that are predictive or provide an early assessment of response with such agents.

4.6 Conclusions

Imaging and tissue biomarkers have become a routine part of the treatment of cancer, and their use will grow with improvements in "omics" (genomics, proteomics, etc.) and imaging technologies. The validation of such markers will remain challenging as we seek to prove that such assays can successfully choose the appropriate therapy and alter the outcome of disease.

References

1 Henry, N.L. and D.F. Hayes, Cancer biomarkers. *Mol Oncol*, 2012. **6**(2): p. 140–146.
2 Hartwell, L., et al., Cancer biomarkers: a systems approach. *Nat Biotechnol*, 2006. **24**(8): p. 905–908.
3 Slamon, D.J., et al., Use of chemotherapy plus a monoclonal antibody against HER2 for metastatic breast cancer that overexpresses HER2. *N Engl J Med*, 2001. **344**(11): p. 783–792.
4 Ratain, M.J., et al., Pharmacodynamics in cancer therapy. *J Clin Oncol*, 1990. **8**(10): p. 1739–1753.
5 Hutter, H., Fluorescent reporter methods. *Methods Mol Biol*, 2006. **351**: p. 155–173.
6 Blasberg, R.G., Imaging update: new windows, new views. *Clin Cancer Res*, 2007. **13**(12): p. 3444–3448.
7 Mankoff, D.A., et al., Tumor-specific positron emission tomography imaging in patients: [18F] fluorodeoxyglucose and beyond. *Clin Cancer Res*, 2007. **13**(12): p. 3460–3469.
8 Mankoff, D.A., et al., Molecular imaging research in the outcomes era: measuring outcomes for individualized cancer therapy. *Acad Radiol*, 2007. **14**(4): p. 398–405.
9 Weber, W.A., Positron emission tomography as an imaging biomarker. *J Clin Oncol*, 2006. **24**(20): p. 3282–3292.
10 Hammond, M.E.H., et al., American Society of Clinical Oncology/College of American Pathologists guideline recommendations for immunohistochemical testing of estrogen and progesterone receptors in breast cancer. *J Clin Oncol*, 2010. **28**(16): p. 2784–2795.
11 Carlson, J.J. and J.A. Roth, The impact of the Oncotype Dx breast cancer assay in clinical practice: a systematic review and meta-analysis. *Breast Cancer Res Treat*, 2013. **141**(1): p. 13–22.
12 Dowsett, M., et al., Assessment of Ki67 in breast cancer: recommendations from the International Ki67 in Breast Cancer working group. *J Natl Cancer Inst*, 2011. **103**(22): p. 1656–1664.
13 DeMichele, A., et al., Developing safety criteria for introducing new agents into neoadjuvant trials. *Clin Cancer Res*, 2013. **19**(11): p. 2817–2823.
14 Welch, D.R., Microarrays bring new insights into understanding of breast cancer metastasis to bone. *Breast Cancer Res*, 2004. **6**(2): p. 61–64.
15 Jakobsen, J.N. and J.B. Sorensen, Clinical impact of ki-67 labeling index in non-small cell lung cancer. *Lung Cancer*, 2013. **79**(1): p. 1–7.
16 Dehdashti, F., et al., Assessing tumor hypoxia in cervical cancer by PET with 60Cu-labeled diacetyl-bis(N4-methylthiosemicarbazone). *J Nucl Med*, 2008. **49**(2): p. 201–205.
17 Wang, W., et al., Prognostic value of [18F]fluorodeoxyglucose positron emission tomographic scanning in patients with thyroid cancer. *J Clin Endocrinol Metab*, 2000. **85**(3): p. 1107–1113.
18 Carr, L.L., et al., Phase II study of daily sunitinib in FDG-PET-positive, iodine-refractory differentiated thyroid cancer and metastatic medullary carcinoma of the thyroid with functional imaging correlation. *Clin Cancer Res*, 2010. **16**(21): p. 5260–5268.
19 Krohn, K.A., J.M. Link, and R.P. Mason, Molecular imaging of hypoxia. *J Nucl Med*, 2008. **49**(Suppl 2): p. 129s–148s.
20 Rajendran, J.G., et al., Tumor hypoxia imaging with [F-18] fluoromisonidazole positron emission tomography in head and neck cancer. *Clin Cancer Res*, 2006. **12**(18): p. 5435–5441.
21 Spence, A.M., et al., Regional hypoxia in glioblastoma multiforme quantified with [18F] fluoromisonidazole positron emission tomography before radiotherapy: correlation with time to progression and survival. *Clin Cancer Res*, 2008. **14**(9): p. 2623–2630.

22 Mankoff, D.A., D.A. Pryma, and A.S. Clark, Molecular imaging biomarkers for oncology clinical trials. *J Nucl Med*, 2014. **55**(4): p. 525–528.

23 Linden, H.M., et al., Quantitative fluoroestradiol positron emission tomography imaging predicts response to endocrine treatment in breast cancer. *J Clin Oncol*, 2006. **24**(18): p. 2793–2799.

24 Mortimer, J.E., et al., Metabolic flare: indicator of hormone responsiveness in advanced breast cancer. *J Clin Oncol*, 2001. **19**(11): p. 2797–2803.

25 Rajendran, J.G., et al., Hypoxia imaging-directed radiation treatment planning. *Eur J Nucl Med Mol Imaging*, 2006. **33**(Suppl 1): p. 44–53.

26 Rischin, D., et al., Prognostic significance of [18F]-misonidazole positron emission tomography-detected tumor hypoxia in patients with advanced head and neck cancer randomly assigned to chemoradiation with or without tirapazamine: a substudy of Trans-Tasman Radiation Oncology Group Study 98.02. *J Clin Oncol*, 2006. **24**(13): p. 2098–2104.

27 Yao, J.C., et al., Everolimus for advanced pancreatic neuroendocrine tumors. *N Engl J Med*, 2011. **364**(6): p. 514–523.

28 Choi, H., et al., Correlation of computed tomography and positron emission tomography in patients with metastatic gastrointestinal stromal tumor treated at a single institution with imatinib mesylate: proposal of new computed tomography response criteria. *J Clin Oncol*, 2007. **25**(13): p. 1753–1759.

29 Weber, J.S., et al., Phase I/II study of ipilimumab for patients with metastatic melanoma. *J Clin Oncol*, 2008. **26**(36): p. 5950–5956.

30 Bading, J.R. and A.F. Shields, Imaging of cell proliferation: status and prospects. *J Nucl Med*, 2008. **49**(Suppl 2): p. 64s–80s.

31 Shields, A.F., et al., Carbon-11-thymidine and FDG to measure therapy response. *J Nucl Med*, 1998. **39**(10): p. 1757–1762.

32 Kenny, L., et al., Imaging early changes in proliferation at 1 week post chemotherapy: a pilot study in breast cancer patients with 3'-deoxy-3'-[18F]fluorothymidine positron emission tomography. *Eur J Nucl Med Mol Imaging*, 2007. **34**(9): p. 1339–1347.

33 Sohn, H.-J., et al., [18F]Fluorothymidine positron emission tomography before and 7 days after gefitinib treatment predicts response in patients with advanced adenocarcinoma of the lung. *Clin Cancer Res*, 2008. **14**(22): p. 7423–7429.

34 Kostakoglu, L., et al., Phase II study of 3'-deoxy-3'-18F fluorothymidine PET/CT (FLT-PET) in the assessment of early response in locally advanced breast cancer (LABC): Preliminary results of ACRIN 6688. *J Clin Oncol*, 2014. **32**(15_suppl): p. 526.

35 Von Hoff, D.D., et al., Increased survival in pancreatic cancer with nab-paclitaxel plus gemcitabine. *N Engl J Med*, 2013. **369**(18): p. 1691–1703.

36 Demetri, G.D., et al., Efficacy and safety of sunitinib in patients with advanced gastrointestinal stromal tumour after failure of imatinib: a randomised controlled trial. *Lancet*, 2006. **368**(9544): p. 1329–1338.

37 Mankoff, D.A., et al., Monitoring the response of patients with locally advanced breast carcinoma to neoadjuvant chemotherapy using [technetium 99m]-sestamibi scintimammography. *Cancer*, 1999. **85**(11): p. 2410–2423.

38 Dunnwald, L.K., et al., Residual tumor uptake of [99mTc]-sestamibi after neoadjuvant chemotherapy for locally advanced breast carcinoma predicts survival. *Cancer*, 2005. **103**(4): p. 680–688.

39 Maini, C.L., et al., Technetium-99m-MIBI scintigraphy in the assessment of neoadjuvant chemotherapy in breast carcinoma. *J Nucl Med*, 1997. **38**(10): p. 1546–1551.

40 Chia, S., et al., Locally advanced and inflammatory breast cancer. *J Clin Oncol*, 2008. **26**(5): p. 786–790.

41 Sargent, D.J., et al., Validation of novel imaging methodologies for use as cancer clinical trial end-points. *Eur J Cancer*, 2009. **45**(2): p. 290–299.

42 McShane, L.M. and D.F. Hayes, Publication of tumor marker research results: the necessity for complete and transparent reporting. *J Clin Oncol*, 2012. **30**(34): p. 4223–4232.

43 Shankar, L.K., et al., Considerations for the use of imaging tools for phase II treatment trials in oncology. *Clin Cancer Res*, 2009. **15**(6): p. 1891–1897.

44 Kostakoglu, L. and B.D. Cheson, State-of-the-art research on "lymphomas: role of molecular imaging for staging, prognostic evaluation, and treatment response". *Front Oncol*, 2013. **3**: p. 212.

45 Gebhart, G., et al., 18F-FDG PET/CT for early prediction of response to neoadjuvant lapatinib, trastuzumab, and their combination in HER2-positive breast cancer: results from Neo-ALTTO. *J Nucl Med*, 2013. **54**(11): p. 1862–1868.

46 Lordick, F., et al., PET to assess early metabolic response and to guide treatment of adenocarcinoma of the oesophagogastric junction: the MUNICON phase II trial. *Lancet Oncol*, 2007. **8**(9): p. 797–805.

47 zum Buschenfelde, C.M., et al., (18)F-FDG PET-guided salvage neoadjuvant radiochemotherapy of adenocarcinoma of the esophagogastric junction: the MUNICON II trial. *J Nucl Med*, 2011. **52**(8): p. 1189–1196.

48 Karapetis, C.S., et al., K-ras mutations and benefit from cetuximab in advanced colorectal cancer. *N Engl J Med*, 2008. **359**(17): p. 1757–1765.

CHAPTER 5

Screening trials and design

Janie M. Lee[1], Constance D. Lehman[1,2] and Diana L. Miglioretti[3]

[1] University of Washington, Boston, MA, USA
[2] Massachusetts General Hospital, Boston, MA, USA
[3] University of California Davis School of Medicine, Davis, CA, USA

KEY POINTS

- Balancing the benefits and harms of screening includes consideration of events within entire screening episodes.

- Important outcomes are condition-specific and multidimensional, extending beyond measurement of mortality reduction.

- Well-designed observational studies and simulation modeling, in addition to randomized trials, are valid study design options for characterizing the benefits, consequences, and outcomes of imaging-based screening.

5.1 Principles of screening

Screening is the systematic testing of asymptomatic individuals to detect a targeted disease. The purpose of screening is to prevent or delay the development of advanced disease through earlier detection and enable less morbid and more effective treatment [1].

This chapter will provide an overview of disease screening and screening trial protocol development, with illustrative examples of recent imaging-based screening studies. When examining a screening program, several factors should be considered: the natural history of the disease of interest, screening test characteristics, and how the screening test and available treatments influence the natural history of disease. When developing a screening trial protocol, critical elements include the identification of the target population, determination of the screening regimens to be compared, and selection of outcomes to be measured and appropriate corresponding study designs.

Handbook for Clinical Trials of Imaging and Image-Guided Interventions, First Edition.
Edited by Nancy A. Obuchowski and G. Scott Gazelle.

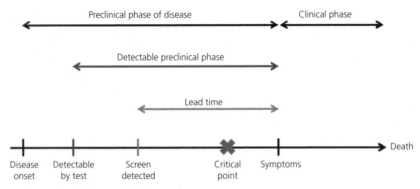

Figure 5.1 Natural history of disease and screening.

5.1.1 Natural history of disease

Screening is usually applied in diseases with serious consequences, both morbidity and mortality [2–4]. Figure 5.1 illustrates the natural history of disease; the first event on the timeline indicates the biologic onset of disease. Disease progresses until symptoms develop and ultimately causes death, unless the individual dies from other causes first. The time interval between the biologic onset of disease and the onset of symptoms represents the **preclinical phase of disease**. Symptomatic presentation marks the onset of the **clinical phase of disease**. The clinically apparent disease will be diagnosed at that time, in the absence of screening, and appropriate treatment initiated. The clinical phase lasts until the death of the patient either from the disease or from other causes.

The interval between when the disease can be identified by the screening test and the development of symptoms is the **detectable preclinical phase of disease**. It marks the window of opportunity for screening to detect disease earlier and enable treatment to improve patient outcomes.

An important event in the natural history of disease is the **critical point**, which identifies the time before which earlier treatment is associated with a better outcome. For example, in the case of cancer, the critical point may be when a cancer metastasizes beyond its primary organ. For screening to be effective in improving patient outcomes, the critical point must occur within the detectable preclinical phase of disease. If the critical point occurs before the detectable preclinical phase, screening would be futile. If the critical point occurs after the disease becomes symptomatic, screening is unnecessary.

Finally, the patient must present for screening if diagnosis of the targeted disease is to occur. The interval between when the disease is detected by screening and when the patient would have presented with clinical signs and symptoms is called the **lead time**.

5.1.2 Screening test characteristics

Screening is distinct from diagnostic testing in that individuals undergoing screening are asymptomatic. The likelihood of disease, or **prevalence**, is substantially lower in asymptomatic patients compared to those with symptoms, which in turn influences the potential impact of a screening program within a population. Because most individuals screened are free of disease, minimizing the potential harms to these individuals and at the same time identifying others with the targeted disease who will benefit from earlier detection and treatment are both critically important aspects of an effective screening program. As a corollary, the prevalence of the targeted disease must be high enough among the individuals screened that commitment of resources to screening would have positive population-level impact.

Important characteristics of any screening test are its sensitivity and specificity [2, 5, 6]. Calculations of these two fundamental measures of diagnostic test performance are based on test result (positive versus negative) and disease status (present versus absent). Individuals with true-positive (TP) test results will have positive screening results, with subsequent work-up resulting in diagnosis of the targeted disease. Those with false-positive (FP) test results will have positive screening results, yet subsequent work-up results will yield a benign diagnosis not targeted by screening. Individuals with true-negative (TN) test results will have negative screening results due to the absence of the targeted disease. In screening, confirmation of TN test results is frequently obtained when no disease is diagnosed during a clinically reasonable follow-up period. Individuals with false-negative (FN) test results will have negative screening results and then subsequently present with clinical signs and symptoms of the targeted disease. **Sensitivity** refers to the proportion of patients with the targeted disease who will have a positive test result, or TP/(TP+FN). **Specificity** represents the proportion of patients without the targeted disease who will have a negative test result, or TN/(TN+FP) (see Chapter 9 for a full description of measures of test accuracy). Reproducibility, safety, availability, and affordability are also test characteristics that will influence the feasibility and success of a screening program [3, 4].

5.2 Screening cascade

A screening intervention extends beyond application of the test itself. Rather, it is an episode of care that begins with the screening test and also includes the subsequent cascade of diagnostic evaluation of positive test results and incidental findings, as well as treatment of the targeted disease. Achieving an overarching balance of benefits and harms with screening includes consideration of events within entire screening episodes (Figure 5.2).

5.2.1 Negative test results
A highly specific screening test, one that correctly excludes patients without the targeted disease, is an essential characteristic of a screening test. Ideally, these patients with TN results will gain reassurance that they do not have the targeted disease from a fast, noninvasive, inexpensive screening test. When the targeted disease is present but the screening test result is negative (FN), the disease will continue to progress until it presents symptomatically, and the patient will not have gained the benefits

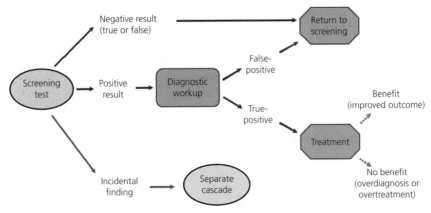

Figure 5.2 Illustration of screening cascade.

of earlier detection with screening. A negative screening test could potentially provide false reassurance and cause an individual to delay seeking care for a symptom, causing further harm.

5.2.2 Positive test results

Because a screening population has no signs or symptoms of disease, it is important to consider the diagnostic consequences of a positive test result [2, 3]. An important potential harm of screening is false-positive results. Individuals with false-positive results will incur all the subsequent diagnostic consequences of a positive test—invasive biopsies, increased costs, and anxiety about having a life-threatening disease—but gain none of the benefits as they did not have the targeted disease [7–10]. The likelihood of having false-positive screening results increases with an increased screening timeframe or with more frequent screening intervals, both of which increase the total number of lifetime screening events, and also with decreasing disease prevalence [11]. Because of these factors, the potential harms of false-positive screening results are most likely to accrue in individuals at lower risk of having the targeted disease. For example, when screening for breast cancer, false-positive results occur more frequently in younger women and decrease as age-specific breast cancer risk increases.

A highly sensitive screening test should detect most patients with the targeted disease (a high TP proportion), enabling earlier disease diagnosis and access to effective treatments. These patients are the ones most likely to obtain the benefits of screening and achieve improved long-term outcomes such as reduced disease-specific mortality.

Even with a highly sensitive test, an important consequence of screening is the potential for harm from overdiagnosis and overtreatment [8, 12, 13]. **Overdiagnosis** and **overtreatment** occur when screening detects asymptomatic disease that would not have become clinically apparent over an individual's lifetime or when screen detection results in treatment of disease that would not have shortened an individual's life expectancy. Both of these scenarios occur more frequently when older populations with higher competing mortality risks undergo screening. Specifically, for cancer, this may be represented by a low-grade malignancy that will not metastasize or cause the patient morbidity or mortality if left alone. Due to the invasive treatment of certain cancers, overdiagnosis and overtreatment may be among the most significant potential harms associated with screening.

5.2.3 Incidental findings

Incidental findings, those discovered during image interpretation that are unrelated to the indication of the study, are a routine part of diagnostic radiology [14]. In examinations with larger fields of view, such as CT when used for lung cancer, colon cancer, or coronary artery disease screening, there is potential for the discovery of multiple incidental findings that are unrelated to the targeted disease. For example, approximately 8% of patients who undergo CT for coronary artery disease screening and 14% of patients who undergo CT for lung cancer screening will have potentially clinically significant incidental findings that require a separate diagnostic work-up [15]. Potential harms from incidental findings may result from complications of unnecessary invasive procedures, increased costs, and undue patient anxiety for what is ultimately determined to be a benign lesion [16]. These "incidentalomas" place patients and their providers in a difficult situation, as it may not be possible to predict which will be clinically significant and which will not at the time of examination interpretation.

5.3 Developing a screening trial protocol

5.3.1 Identify the target population

It is essential to identify an appropriate population of patients to undergo screening so that the benefits of screening will accrue for patients with the targeted disease and potential harms can be minimized for patients without disease. Important patient characteristics to specify include age range, gender, and additional risk factors for disease. For example, the United States Preventive Services Task Force (USPSTF) recommends low-dose CT screening for lung cancer in asymptomatic adults aged 55–80 years who have a 30-pack-year smoking history and currently smoke or have quit within the past 15 years [17].

5.3.2 Determine the screening regimens to be compared

Comparative effectiveness research (CER) has emerged as an important approach for providing high-value, cost-conscious health care. CER focuses on answering real-world questions about "what works for which patients under what circumstances" [18–21]. For screening studies, where a large number of asymptomatic patients are screened to identify the relative few who will benefit, an important aspect of study design will involve determining appropriate comparators for a new screening test. While comparison with "no screening" is best to demonstrate that a new screening test is effective at reducing morbidity and/or mortality of disease, comparing the new test with currently available options for screening of the targeted disease will provide a clearer determination of its achievable benefits. For example, in the National Lung Screening Trial (NLST) of low-dose CT, chest radiography was chosen as the screening method for the control group [22]. Additional considerations in selecting a screening regimen for evaluation include whether a screening test will be used alone or in conjunction with other screening tests (such as mammography and MRI for screening BRCA mutation carriers [23]), the screening interval (annually, biennially, or other), and ages for patients to begin and end screening.

5.3.3 Select clinical efficacy goals

Once the appropriate patient population and screening regimens have been determined, the next step in developing a screening trial protocol involves assessing the critical knowledge gaps related to the screening test and its effect on patient outcomes, or clinical efficacy. In Chapter 1 we described a hierarchical model for understanding the clinical efficacy of diagnostic imaging, with efficacy at lower levels required before efficacy at higher levels can be achieved [24]. This organizing framework can also guide selection of efficacy goals and study design for a trial evaluating a new screening test.

When a clinical trial of imaging screening is being considered, technical efficacy has usually been achieved, with high-quality images consistently being produced. The next level of clinical efficacy to be evaluated is that of diagnostic accuracy and diagnostic thinking (see Chapter 1). The higher levels involve clinical efficacy, therapeutic efficacy, patient outcome, and societal efficacy. Studies of diagnostic accuracy and efficacy also frequently include a component focused on therapeutic efficacy, such as reporting changes in surrogate outcomes. For example, when mammography is used to screen for breast cancer, screen-detected breast cancers are smaller in size and less likely to involve axillary lymph nodes [25]. Breast cancer diagnosis at earlier stages with screening has been shown to be an excellent surrogate for the longer-term outcome of reduced breast cancer-specific mortality with mammographic screening [26], as shown in multiple randomized trials [27, 28].

When evaluating longer-term patient outcomes, two endpoints to consider are survival versus mortality [2, 29]. At first glance, mortality and survival would seem to be complementary endpoints with proportions that sum to one. However, one should measure survival with caution, as comparisons of survival are more prone to bias, compared with disease-specific mortality or overall mortality (see Chapter 10 for more details).

Lead time, length time, and overdiagnosis/overtreatment biases all favor screening and should be minimized where possible in study design and analysis. **Lead time bias** can be observed when survival is measured from the time of diagnosis and screening results in earlier detection of the targeted disease. Even if screening is ineffective, the addition of lead time to measurements of survival results in an apparent increase in life expectancy attributed to screening. **Length time bias** can make screening appear more effective because screening tests preferentially detect disease that progresses more slowly and has a longer detectable preclinical phase. The extreme form of length time bias is overdiagnosis and overtreatment (see Section 5.2.2).

When considering disease-specific versus overall mortality as a primary endpoint for a screening study, disease-specific mortality is the most widely used outcome measure for a screening test. It is important to note that use of this endpoint relies on the assumption that the cause of death can be determined accurately. In addition, it can underestimate the potential harms of screening by failing to identify any possible increased mortality associated with treatment of the detected disease. Overall mortality is an endpoint that is not affected by cause-of-death misclassification. It also puts the effect of screening in the context of overall population mortality. However, overall mortality is an insensitive measure of screening efficacy and requires much larger and potentially infeasible sample sizes to demonstrate a statistically significant benefit from screening. Because both these mortality endpoints are complementary, it is useful to evaluate both of them. The NLST reported relative reductions of 20% for lung cancer-specific mortality and 7% for overall mortality attributable to low-dose CT screening [22].

Additional outcomes of interest such as radiation-induced cancer mortality, life years gained, or deaths averted by screening cannot be directly measured in a clinical trial. These outcome measures can be projected using computer simulation modeling, which uses quantitative methods to integrate short-term evidence about diagnostic tests and treatments to project longer-term outcomes [30, 31]. Simulation modeling can also project outcomes that are not otherwise available and are frequently of interest to policy makers. An example of simulation modeling to inform screening guidelines is the Cancer Intervention and Surveillance Modeling Network's (CISNET) evaluation of multiple potential screening regimens not included in randomized clinical trials to guide USPSTF recommendations for colorectal, breast, and lung cancer screening [32–34]. Simulation modeling has also been used to evaluate societal efficacy, such as the cost-effectiveness of mammography and MRI for screening BRCA gene mutation carriers [35, 36] (see Chapter 11).

5.3.4 Balance the benefits and potential harms of screening

The burden of proof for the effectiveness of screening is higher than that for diagnostic tests and treatments. Of all the individuals who will undergo screening, those with TP test results who receive effective treatment and are not overdiagnosed will obtain the primary benefits of screening, which include decreased morbidity and mortality related to the targeted disease and its treatment [2]. As we increasingly focus on providing value-based health care, with the goal of improving patient outcomes while maintaining or decreasing health-care costs [37], the important outcomes to measure extend beyond those of mortality reduction. Outcomes that matter are condition-specific and multidimensional—no single outcome will capture the effects of screening. Implementation of new imaging-based screening tests in clinical practice will increasingly hinge on the successful conduct of research on a scale and with a level of rigor not seen in the past [38].

The challenge and opportunity for future research studies of imaging-based screening are to provide evidence on multiple outcomes to characterize not only its benefits but also its downstream consequences and potential harms. Improved quality of life (QoL) or reduced disease-specific mortality must be considered in the context of radiation-induced risks, utilization of additional resources to evaluate incidental findings, false-positive test results, and the potential for overdiagnosis and overtreatment. The budget impact and cost-effectiveness of screening are also important factors requiring examination before adoption and implementation of a new screening program (see Chapter 11).

5.4 Selecting a study design

5.4.1 Randomized controlled trials

Randomized controlled trials (RCTs) are widely considered the best method to obtain evidence on the effectiveness of screening [29, 39]. The primary strength of an RCT is the intention of even distribution of known and unknown confounders across intervention arms of the trial. Thus, observed differences in outcomes can be attributed to differences in intervention (see Chapter 7).

However, not all RCTs are of equal quality, and RCTs have important limitations [40, 41]. RCTs can suffer from pitfalls such as biased randomization or contamination, which occurs when individuals randomized to the control arm receive the new screening test or when those offered the new screening test do not receive it. These pitfalls can influence study results when study arms are analyzed based on study arm assignment. RCTs may be limited in terms of generalizability, as they frequently have restrictive inclusion criteria so that study patients are not representative of patients seen in clinical practice, especially with regard to comorbidities, race and ethnicity, or socioeconomic status. RCTs of screening may not be feasible due to their requirements for large sample sizes to demonstrate a statistically significant effect of screening, follow-up on the order of years or decades to determine outcomes, and associated costs.

To guide health-care policy decisions, robust high-quality evidence is needed both about **clinical efficacy** (how a test or treatment performs under ideal conditions) and **clinical effectiveness** (how a test or treatment performs in settings where it will be applied). RCTs focusing on efficacy have also been described as "**explanatory**," while those focusing on effectiveness have been described as "**pragmatic**" [42]. To assist clinical trialists in making study design decisions that meet their study aims, the pragmatic–explanatory continuum indicator summary (PRECIS) tool contains 10 domains related to clinical trial design and produces a graphical summary of where a trial's design falls on the explanatory-to-pragmatic spectrum [43].

5.4.2 Observational studies

The emergence of comparative effectiveness research has led to a renewed interest in observational studies as an alternative to RCTs for assessing the effects of tests and treatments [29, 39, 44]. Observational studies differ from RCTs by comparing outcomes in groups receiving different interventions, which are assigned by a process other than randomization. This may be due to patient characteristics that result in exposure to different interventions or factors external to the patient such as provider characteristics or policy changes that result in different groups of patients receiving different interventions. Observational studies may be prospective or retrospective, and designs include correlation, case–control, and cohort studies. Strengths of observational studies include the ability to study more diverse patient populations compared with RCTs, larger sample sizes due to less restrictive inclusion criteria, and performance in both community and academic settings, making these study results more generalizable to broader practice settings.

Observational studies also have limitations, such as being more subject to bias (see Chapter 7 for additional biases common in imaging studies). **Selection bias** occurs when screened individuals are at different risk for the targeted disease compared with unscreened individuals. The direction of bias can vary—if the risk is higher in those receiving screening, then selection bias will be against screening, whereas if the risk is lower in those receiving screening, then selection bias will favor screening. Retrospective observational studies are prone to **observer bias** on the part of investigators abstracting data and to **recall bias** on the part of patients reporting their screening exposures. Finally, observational studies can be subject to **confounding**, in which differences are present between screened and control groups, which are also related to the outcomes of interest. While statistical adjustment for known confounders can be performed, the effects of unknown confounders will remain.

5.4.3 Role of computer simulation modeling

As discussed earlier, computer simulation modeling can be a powerful tool to project outcomes that cannot be directly measured in clinical trials. This methodology may also be used to extrapolate the results of clinical trials to settings where population characteristics, methods of screening, screening intervals, and other factors differ from those included clinical trials.

5.4.4 Illustrative examples of imaging-based screening trials

This section provides examples of imaging-based screening trials with varying endpoints, study designs, and secondary aims, as well as discussion of the impact of these trials. We will consider three trials conducted by the American College of Radiology Imaging Network (ACRIN): digital mammography for breast cancer screening, CT colonography (CTC) for colorectal cancer screening, and low-dose CT for lung cancer screening.

Digital Mammographic Imaging Screening Trial (DMIST) [45]: DMIST was a diagnostic accuracy trial designed to measure relatively small but potentially clinically important differences in diagnostic accuracy between digital and film mammography. The study used a prospective cohort observational design. During a 2-year period, 49,528 women were recruited to the study at 33 sites. Women who presented for screening mammography at the study sites underwent both digital and film mammography in random order, with examinations for each woman independently interpreted by two radiologists. Diagnostic work-up was performed if either test had a positive result. Either pathology diagnosis of breast cancer or a negative follow-up mammogram a year later was used to determine the presence or absence of breast cancer. Receiver Operating Characteristic (ROC) analysis was used to evaluate the results.

The trial results indicated that the diagnostic accuracy of digital and film mammography was similar, with a nonsignificant difference in area under their respective ROC curves. However, the accuracy of digital mammography was significantly higher for some subgroups of women: those under 50 years of age, those with heterogeneously or extremely dense breasts, or premenopausal women. Publication of the DMIST results was associated with a steep increase in the adoption of digital mammography. While the prevalence of digital mammography units was less than 10% of all units at the time of study publication in 2005, less than a decade later, approximately 95% of accredited mammography units in the United States were digital [46].

DMIST also included evaluation of quality of life and cost-effectiveness as secondary aims. The DMIST QoL study of 1028 women [9] included two groups: (i) a random sample of DMIST participants with false-positive screening results and (ii) a sample of women with negative screening mammograms matched by study site and age. Patient anxiety and health utility (quality of life rated on a scale of 0–100, with 0 representing death and 100 representing perfect health) were measured using validated instruments. Telephone surveys were conducted at baseline and approximately 1 year later.

The QoL results indicated that having an false-positive screening mammogram result was associated with significantly increased anxiety that resolved within 1 year, with no measurable decrease in quality of life. In multivariable analyses, women in either group who reported feeling high anxiety about future false-positive screening results expressed a greater willingness to travel up to 4 hours to avoid having such a result (OR 1.94, 95% CI 1.28–2.95). The investigators concluded that evidence of women's motivation to avoid false-positive screening results, regardless of whether they actually received them, would be useful information for health-care providers who counsel individual women about breast cancer screening and for policy makers assessing the clinical effectiveness of mammographic screening.

The DMIST QoL study results were also used to calculate economic time costs of follow-up diagnostic testing after a positive screening mammography result. These costs were incorporated into a cost-effectiveness analysis [10], which indicated that, compared with film mammography, digital mammography was more cost-effective when its use was guided by patient age rather than broad use across all women. The age-targeted digital mammography screening strategy for women less than 50 years of age projected costs of $26,500 to gain an additional quality-adjusted life year (QALY), while all-women use of digital mammography would cost $331,000 per QALY gained.

A subsequent simulation modeling study by the CISNET breast group [47] supported these initial estimates, reporting that the transition to digital mammography screening in the United States increased total breast cancer screening costs for small added health benefits. Further, they reported that the value of digital mammography screening among women aged 40–49 years depends on women's preferences regarding FP test results. Current efforts to improve mammography screening outcomes are focused on combining patient age with additional risk factors such as breast density and family history to guide more tailored selection of screening initiation age and screening interval for individual patients [48, 49].

National CT Colonography Trial [50]: This trial was designed to assess the diagnostic accuracy of CTC in detecting histologically confirmed, large colorectal adenomas and cancers (≥10 mm in diameter). The study used a prospective cohort observational design, recruiting 2531 asymptomatic study participants, 50 years of age or older, at 15 study sites. Radiologists trained in CTC interpretation reported all lesions measuring 5 mm or more in diameter. Optical colonoscopy, the alternative clinical standard for colorectal cancer screening, was subsequently performed. Colonoscopy and histologic review served as the reference standard. The primary endpoint was CTC detection of histologically confirmed large adenomas and adenocarcinomas (10 mm in diameter or larger) that had been detected by colonoscopy; detection of smaller colorectal lesions (6–9 mm in diameter) was also evaluated. The study reported sensitivity of CTC to be 0.90 with specificity of 0.86 and area under the ROC curve of 0.89 for detecting large adenomas and cancers.

The National CT Colonography Trial diagnostic accuracy results were included in a CISNET study using simulation modeling to evaluate alternative colorectal cancer screening options for the Medicare population of US adults aged 65 and older [51]. Its results indicated that CTC performed at 5-year intervals was less effective than colonoscopy performed at 10-year intervals and that CTC could be cost-effective if the reimbursement rate per scan was substantially less than that for colonoscopy or if a large proportion of otherwise unscreened individuals were to undergo screening by CTC. This information was cited by CMS in its decision of noncoverage for CTC for colorectal cancer screening in the Medicare population [52]. A subsequent cost-effectiveness analysis of CTC based on National CT Colonography Trial data also concluded that CTC was more costly and less effective than non-CT colonographic screening. When screening strategies were ranked by net health benefits, a measure of economic efficiency, CTC strategies had lower net benefits compared with sigmoidoscopy and colonoscopy strategies and higher net benefits when compared with no screening [53]. Currently, most third-party payers provide reimbursement for screening CTC only after a failed optical colonoscopy or, in some cases, for individuals who have a contraindication to colonoscopy [54].

National Lung Screening Trial (NLST) [22]: This trial was conducted to determine whether screening with low-dose CT could reduce mortality from lung cancer. Using an RCT design, the NLST enrolled 53,454 men and women at 33 US medical centers. Eligible participants were between 55 and 74 years of age at the time of randomization, had a history of cigarette smoking of at least 30 pack-years, and, if former smokers, had quit within the previous 15 years. Participants were randomly assigned to undergo three annual screenings with either low-dose CT (*n* = 26,722) or chest radiography (*n* = 26,732). Data were subsequently collected on cases of lung cancer and deaths from lung cancer. Death certificates were obtained for participants who were known to have died. An endpoint verification team blinded to screening arm assignment determined whether or not an individual's cause of death was lung cancer.

The study reported results of a relative reduction in mortality from lung cancer with low-dose CT screening of 20.0% (95% CI, 6.8–26.7; $P = 0.004$). The rate of death from any cause was reduced in the low-dose CT group, as compared with the radiography group, by 6.7% (95% CI, 1.2–13.6; $P = 0.02$). A subsequent NLST publication reported on the diagnostic accuracy of lung cancer screening tests [55]. Sensitivity and specificity were 94 and 73% for low-dose CT and 74 and 91% for chest radiography, respectively.

This CISNET lung group calibrated its simulation models to reproduce the lung cancer incidence and mortality outcomes of the NLST and another lung cancer screening trial, the Prostate, Lung, Colorectal and Ovarian Cancer Screening Trial [56]. The models were then used to evaluate 576 potential screening regimens with varying eligibility criteria (age, pack-years of smoking, years since quitting) and screening intervals [32]. The modeling results indicated that annual CT screening for lung cancer has a favorable benefit–harm ratio for individuals aged 55 through 80 years with 30 or more pack-years' exposure to smoking. With this strategy, 50% of cases of lung cancer would be detected at an early stage (stage I or II). In addition, for every 100,000 individuals screened, lung cancer mortality would be reduced by 14%, 497 lung cancer deaths would be averted, and 5250 life years would be gained. Harms would include 67,550 FP test results, 910 biopsies or surgeries for benign lesions, and 190 overdiagnosed cases of cancer (3.7% of all cases of lung cancer). In its 2014 recommendations supporting low-dose CT for lung cancer screening, USPSTF concluded "with moderate certainty that annual screening for lung cancer with low-dose CT is of moderate net benefit in asymptomatic persons who are at high risk for lung cancer based on age, total cumulative exposure to tobacco smoke, and years since quitting smoking" [17].

References

1 Hillman, B.J., et al., The appropriateness of employing imaging screening technologies: report of the methods committee of the ACR task force on screening technologies. *J Am Coll Radiol*, 2004. **1**(11): p. 861–864.

2 Black, W.C. and H.G. Welch, Screening for disease. *AJR Am J Roentgenol*, 1997. **168**(1): p. 3–11.

3 Obuchowski, N.A., et al., Ten criteria for effective screening: their application to multislice CT screening for pulmonary and colorectal cancers. *AJR Am J Roentgenol*, 2001. **176**(6): p. 1357–1362.

4 Wilson, J. and G. Jungner, *Principles and Practice of Screening for Disease*, 1968, World Health Organization: Geneva.

5 Weinstein, S., N.A. Obuchowski, and M.L. Lieber, Clinical evaluation of diagnostic tests. *AJR Am J Roentgenol*, 2005. **184**(1): p. 14–19.

6 Langlotz, C.P., Fundamental measures of diagnostic examination performance: usefulness for clinical decision making and research. *Radiology*, 2003. **228**(1): p. 3–9.

7 Brewer, N.T., T. Salz, and S.E. Lillie, Systematic review: the long-term effects of false-positive mammograms. *Ann Intern Med*, 2007. **146**(7): p. 502–510.

8 Harris, R.P., et al., The harms of screening: a proposed taxonomy and application to lung cancer screening. *JAMA Intern Med*, 2014. **174**(2): p. 281–285.

9 Tosteson, A.N., et al., Consequences of false-positive screening mammograms. *JAMA Intern Med*, 2014. **174**(6): p. 954–961.

10 Tosteson, A.N., et al., Cost-effectiveness of digital mammography breast cancer screening. *Ann Intern Med*, 2008. **148**(1): p. 1–10.

11 Hubbard, R.A., et al., Cumulative probability of false-positive recall or biopsy recommendation after 10 years of screening mammography: a cohort study. *Ann Intern Med*, 2011. **155**(8): p. 481–492.

12 Esserman, L., Y. Shieh, and I. Thompson, Rethinking screening for breast cancer and prostate cancer. *JAMA*, 2009. **302**(15): p. 1685–1692.

13 Welch, H.G. and W.C. Black, Overdiagnosis in cancer. *J Natl Cancer Inst*, 2010. **102**(9): p. 605–613.

14 Brown, S.D., Professional norms regarding how radiologists handle incidental findings. *J Am Coll Radiol*, 2013. **10**(4): p. 253–257.

15 Jacobs, P.C.A., et al., Prevalence of incidental findings in computed tomographic screening of the chest: a systematic review. *J Comput Assist Tomogr*, 2008. **32**(2): p. 214–221.

16 Ding, A., J.D. Eisenberg, and P.V. Pandharipande, The economic burden of incidentally detected findings. *Radiol Clin North Am*, 2011. **49**(2): p. 257–265.

17 Moyer, V.A., Screening for lung cancer: U.S. Preventive Services Task Force recommendation statement. *Ann Intern Med*, 2014. **160**(5): p. 330–338.

18 Gazelle GS, et al., A framework for assessing the value of diagnostic imaging in the era of comparative effectiveness research. *Radiology*, 2011. **261**(3): p. 692–698.

19 National Research Council, *Initial National Priorities for Comparative Effectiveness Research*. 2009, The National Academies Press: Washington, DC. p. 252.

20 Owens, D.K., et al., High-value, cost-conscious health care: concepts for clinicians to evaluate the benefits, harms, and costs of medical interventions. *Ann Intern Med*, 2011. **154**(3): p. 174–180.

21 Federal Coordinating Council for Comparative Effectiveness Research, *Report to the President and the Congress, June 30, 2009*. 2009, United States Department of Health and Human Services: Washington, DC.

22 National Lung Screening Trial Research Team, et al., Reduced lung-cancer mortality with low-dose computed tomographic screening. *N Engl J Med*, 2011. **365**(5): p. 395–409.

23 Saslow, D., et al., American Cancer Society guidelines for breast screening with MRI as an adjunct to mammography. *CA Cancer J Clin*, 2007. **57**(2): p. 75–89.

24 Fryback, D.G. and J.R. Thornbury, The efficacy of diagnostic imaging. *Med Decis Making*, 1991. **11**(2): p. 88–94.

25 Swedish Organised Service Screening Evaluation Group, Effect of mammographic service screening on stage at presentation of breast cancers in Sweden. *Cancer*, 2007. **109**(11): p. 2205–2212.

26 Smart, C.R., et al., Twenty-year follow-up of the breast cancers diagnosed during the Breast Cancer Detection Demonstration Project. *CA Cancer J Clin*, 1997. **47**(3): p. 134–149.

27 Nelson, H.D., et al., Screening for breast cancer: an update for the U.S. Preventive Services Task Force. *Ann Intern Med*, 2009. **151**(10): p. 727–737.

28 Tabar, L., et al., Swedish two-county trial: impact of mammographic screening on breast cancer mortality during 3 decades. *Radiology*, 2011. **260**(3): p. 658–663.

29 Black, W.C., Randomized clinical trials for cancer screening: rationale and design considerations for imaging tests. *J Clin Oncol*, 2006. **24**(20): p. 3252–3260.

30 Kong, C.Y., et al., Using radiation risk models in cancer screening simulations: important assumptions and effects on outcome projections. *Radiology*, 2012. **262**(3): p. 977–984.

31 Rutter, C.M., A.B. Knudsen, and P.V. Pandharipande, Computer disease simulation models: integrating evidence for health policy. *Acad Radiol*, 2011. **18**(9): p. 1077–1086.

32 Zauber, A.G., et al., Evaluating test strategies for colorectal cancer screening: a decision analysis for the U.S. Preventive Services Task Force. *Ann Intern Med*, 2008. **149**(9): p. 659–669.

33 Mandelblatt, J.S., et al., Effects of mammography screening under different screening schedules: model estimates of potential benefits and harms. *Ann Intern Med*, 2009. **151**(10): p. 738–747.

34 de Koning, H.J., et al., Benefits and harms of computed tomography lung cancer screening strategies: a comparative modeling study for the U.S. Preventive Services Task Force. *Ann Intern Med*, 2014. **160**(5): p. 311–320.

35 Plevritis, S.K., et al., Cost-effectiveness of screening BRCA1/2 mutation carriers with breast magnetic resonance imaging. *JAMA*, 2006. **295**(20): p. 2374–2384.

36 Cott Chubiz, J.E., et al., Cost-effectiveness of alternating magnetic resonance imaging and digital mammography screening in BRCA1 and BRCA2 gene mutation carriers. *Cancer*, 2013. **119**(6): p. 1266–1276.

37 Porter, M.E., What is value in health care? *N Engl J Med*, 2010. **363**(26): p. 2477–2481.

38 Thrall, J.H., Building research programs in diagnostic radiology. Part III. Clinical and translational research. *Radiology*, 2007. **243**(1): p. 5–9.

39 Armstrong, K., Methods in comparative effectiveness research. *J Clin Oncol*, 2012. **30**(34): p. 4208–4214.

40 Benson, K. and A.J. Hartz, A comparison of observational studies and randomized, controlled trials. *N Engl J Med*, 2000. **342**(25): p. 1878–1886.

41 Concato, J., N. Shah, and R.I. Horwitz, Randomized, controlled trials, observational studies, and the hierarchy of research designs. *N Engl J Med*, 2000. **342**(25): p. 1887–1892.

42 Tunis, S.R., D.B. Stryer, and C.M. Clancy, Practical clinical trials: increasing the value of clinical research for decision making in clinical and health policy. *JAMA*, 2003. **290**(12): p. 1624–1632.

43 Thorpe, K.E., et al., A pragmatic-explanatory continuum indicator summary (PRECIS): a tool to help trial designers. *J Clin Epidemiol*, 2009. **62**(5): p. 464–475.

44 Dreyer, N.A., et al., Why observational studies should be among the tools used in comparative effectiveness research. *Health Aff (Millwood)*, 2010. **29**(10): p. 1818–1825.

45 Pisano, E., et al., Diagnostic performance of digital versus film mammography for breast-cancer screening. *N Engl J Med*, 2005. **353**(17): p. 1773–1783.

46 United States Food and Drug Administration, Mammography Quality Standards Act National Statistics. 2014; Available from: http://www.fda.gov/Radiation-EmittingProducts/MammographyQualityStandardsActandProgram/FacilityScorecard/ucm113858.htm (accessed June 7, 2014).

47 Stout, N.K., et al., Benefits, harms, and costs for breast cancer screening after US implementation of digital mammography. *J Natl Cancer Inst*, 2014. **106**(6): p. dju092.

48 Schousboe, J.T., et al., Personalizing mammography by breast density and other risk factors for breast cancer: analysis of health benefits and cost-effectiveness. *Ann Intern Med*, 2011. **155**(1): p. 10–20.

49 van Ravesteyn, N.T., et al., Tipping the balance of benefits and harms to favor screening mammography starting at age 40 years: a comparative modeling study of risk. *Ann Intern Med*, 2012. **156**(9): p. 609–617.

50 Johnson, C.D., et al., Accuracy of CT colonography for detection of large adenomas and cancers. *N Engl J Med*, 2008. **359**(12): p. 1207–1217.

51 Knudsen, A.B., et al., Cost-effectiveness of computed tomographic colonography screening for colorectal cancer in the medicare population. *J Natl Cancer Inst*, 2010. **102**(16): p. 1238–1252.

52 Centers for Medicare and Medicaid Services, *Decision Memo for Screening Computed Tomography Colonography (CTC) for Colorectal Cancer (CAG-00396N)*. 2009, Washington, DC.

53 Vanness, D.J., et al., Comparative economic evaluation of data from the ACRIN National CT Colonography Trial with three cancer intervention and surveillance modeling network microsimulations. *Radiology*, 2011. **261**(2): p. 487–498.

54 Yee, J., et al., ACR Appropriateness Criteria colorectal cancer screening. *J Am Coll Radiol*, 2014. **11**(6): p. 543–551.

55 Church, T.R., et al., Results of initial low-dose computed tomographic screening for lung cancer. *N Engl J Med*, 2013. **368**(21): p. 1980–1991.

56 Meza, R., et al., Comparative analysis of 5 lung cancer natural history and screening models that reproduce outcomes of the NLST and PLCO trials. *Cancer*, 2014. **120**(11): p. 1713–1724.

CHAPTER 6

Practicalities of running a clinical trial

Michael T. Lu, Elizabeth C. Adami and Udo Hoffmann

Massachusetts General Hospital & Harvard Medical School, Boston, MA, USA

KEY POINTS

- Engaging in clinical research can be very exciting if thought of as a career of highly innovative and significant contributions to improved care for patients.
- Choice of topics should be guided by an experienced mentor and tailored to the investigators' experience and the institutional environment.
- There are many operational and regulatory aspects of research that should be addressed prospectively with a defined set of operational skills and setups.

In this chapter we provide advice on whether and what kind of clinical trial to pursue and practical pointers and common pitfalls of running a clinical trial and recount our experiences with a number of different trials from both the perspective of a principal investigator (PI) and a project manager. Throughout the chapter we will use our own experiences primarily with clinical trials from the area of cardiovascular imaging, specifically the journey of coronary computed tomography angiography (CCTA) from a new tool in 2001 to an established diagnostic test. These practical tips can easily be applied to other imaging techniques.

6.1 Types of clinical trials

In Chapter 1 we discussed different types of research questions and the corresponding hierarchy of clinical trials assessing imaging modalities. In Table 6.1 we use the hierarchical framework of Gazelle [1] to describe the assessment of CCTA. "Hierarchy" implies an ordinal relationship—the higher-order trials of

---

Handbook for Clinical Trials of Imaging and Image-Guided Interventions, First Edition.
Edited by Nancy A. Obuchowski and G. Scott Gazelle.
© 2016 John Wiley & Sons, Inc. Published 2016 by John Wiley & Sons, Inc.

Table 6.1 Assessment hierarchy for CCTA.

Technical performance: Can CCTA be performed to provide high-resolution, motion-free images of the coronary arteries?

Diagnostic accuracy: Does CCTA allow for an accurate clinical diagnosis compared with the reference standard (in this case invasive coronary angiography (ICA))?

Impact on diagnostic thinking: Can CCTA be an effective replacement for ICA for the diagnosis of coronary artery disease?

Impact on therapeutic planning: Can unique findings visible only on CCTA allow for a change in therapeutic planning?

Patient health outcomes: Does the use of CCTA result in improved downstream health outcomes, such as mortality, major adverse cardiac events, and radiation exposure?

Costs and benefits to society: On a population basis, is the use of CCTA cost-effective?

increasing complexity and generalizability require a solid foundation of early phase studies. While imaging tests are often quickly adopted for a new clinical application, the larger hurdle of widespread acceptance and reimbursement is tied to "evidence-based medicine" or, in lack thereof, to appropriateness criteria and societal guidelines based on expert opinion. The highest level of evidence is delivered by multicenter randomized clinical trials demonstrating the superiority of the new strategy (e.g., CT colonography, CCTA, and CT lung cancer screening) as compared to the previous standard of care. This is not to say that trials lower on the hierarchy have less value—in fact they are necessary steps to bringing a new imaging test into practice, and many illustrious careers have been made based on studies of diagnostic accuracy. However in this chapter, we will focus on the third, fourth, and fifth levels of Table 6.1, which go beyond accuracy and are necessary to establish a diagnostic test in clinical practice.

6.2 Practical issues in designing a clinical trial

The reality is that it is totally impractical to run a clinical trial. It is far more convenient to base your practice on anecdotal observations or a review of small retrospective case series. A prospective clinical trial requires substantially more effort, time, and money. This usually means you will need to persuade an organization such as the National Institutes of Health (NIH) or an industry sponsor to fund the trial. You must have the persuasiveness and fortitude to convince your colleagues to do and tolerate something that otherwise would not be done. As the trial may cause harm to your research subjects, the regulatory and institutional review board (IRB) hurdles you must surmount are far higher. You will stake your professional reputation on the outcome of the trial, and you will worry about patient safety, the accuracy of your data, the significance of your results, and how they will impact your ability to obtain future grants.

It is important to make the process as practical and enjoyable as possible. Clinical trials are worth doing because they are innovative and significant. Innovation comes from bringing new fields together by looking for an application of a test that is different than initially thought of. Significance comes from the high impact of the trial—in today's environment of "evidence-based" medicine, payers such as the Centers for Medicare and Medicaid Services are only willing to pay for imaging tests with proven benefit. The burden of proof required is most often several multicenter randomized controlled trials that prove efficacy and cost-effectiveness over the status quo. The study may address inferences of current medical practice or a controversial practice. In short, there are many reasons why you, your colleagues, and ultimately your research subjects should be excited enough to devote time to the trial.

> Remember that Time is Money. He that can earn Ten Shillings a Day by his Labour, and goes abroad, or sits idle one half of that Day, tho' he spends but Sixpence during his Diversion or Idleness, ought not to reckon That the only Expence; he has really spent or rather thrown away Five Shillings besides. Advice to a Young Tradesman, Written by an Old One; Benjamin Franklin [2].

Benjamin Franklin's maxim "time is money" certainly applies to clinical trials. Not only are clinical trials expensive, but also they will require a great deal of your and your colleagues' time that could be spent elsewhere. Costs include personnel, equipment, patient care costs, imaging costs, IRB costs, and contracting costs. Budgeting is addressed in greater detail later in this chapter, but when justifying your budget to the granting agency, you should write down what you expect from everybody and their responsibilities. Make a realistic budget—then go to your chairman and make sure it is realistic. No matter the funding agency, buy-in from your institution is critical for a number of reasons. The NIH salary cap may not be sufficient to pay your institution's salary, in-kind resources such as scanner time may be negotiable, and invariably issues will come up during the course of the trial where having the support of your department and, if applicable, other departments at your institution will be invaluable.

6.2.1 Do the right trial

Take stock of your institution and your situation. What stage of your career are you at? How much experience do you have, or more specifically what experience do you have in this particular area? Do you have a strong mentor and departmental support for your idea? Do you have strong collaborations in areas where you are not an expert? Is the study feasible? Do you have access to the necessary equipment? Do you have a sufficient pool of subjects and the means to recruit

Table 6.2 Considerations in conducting a clinical trial.

Consideration	Definition	How to
Significance	High impact (affects many people)	Run ideas by your colleagues and mentors
	Addresses inefficiencies of current medical practice or a controversial practice	Present in an official forum (lab meeting)
Innovation	Brings new fields together	Collaborations with colleagues outside your specialty
	Applies a test in a field that is different than initially thought of	Attend meetings outside your field
Feasibility	Expertise, technology, patient populations, support	Tailor complexity of the study to these factors
		Check for patient availability in hospital databases
		Talk to your chairman about support
Budget	Personnel, equipment, patient care costs, IRB	Check different funding sources: societies, industry, NIH, hospital, foundations
		Budget time for investigators appropriately
		Write your budget justification as you are writing the grant
		Incentivize sites and investigators sufficiently (at least 2/3 of the budget should be spent on sites/patients)
		Check with clinical investigators to gauge what is appropriate amount of effort
		Account for regular expenses that are often forgotten: materials/supplies, shipping costs, software license fees, expansion drives, replacement PCs for long studies
Enrollment and outcomes	Study protocol and MOP	Regular meeting and review of milestones
	Site training and certification	Predefined rules for situations when falling behind
	Enrollment projections and milestones	Have a point person
	Declining sites and dealing with problem sites	Website on shared experiences to maintain enthusiasm and momentum
	Recruitment slower than anticipated	Interim analysis and QA
	Outcomes rarer than anticipated	Approach a sponsor for additional funds or an extension
Publication and dissemination of results	Publication committee Charter	Schedule of abstracts, publications, and press releases

them efficiently? Ultimately you must match the complexity of your trial to yourself and the environment.

6.2.2 Define trial complexity

You must anticipate the administrative, operational, and ethical challenges to performing the study compliant with good medical practice and regulations (IRB, FDA, etc.). Generally speaking, complexity increases from:

- Retrospective to prospective design
- Cross-section to outcome trial
- Single to multicenter trial
- Nonrandomized to randomized
- Small to large number of subjects
- Healthier to sicker subjects
- Unblinded to blinded readers
- Single to multimodality design

Other considerations that will be helpful to execute a clinical research idea are given in Table 6.2.

6.3 Case of CCTA

Technological advances offer unique opportunities to perform innovative and significant research. For example, 15 years ago the only way to assess for coronary artery stenosis was by invasive coronary angiography (ICA). In 1999/2000 multi-slice CT provided sufficient initial evidence that it would be capable of noninvasively assessing for coronary artery disease (CAD). This was not only novel but for sure a game changer as more than 10 million patients are presenting each year with suspicion for CAD and there was no other tool in sight as a competitor. In this scenario, even small accuracy studies are significant. From 2000 to 2004, we and others performed small, prospective, single-center, blinded accuracy studies to determine the diagnostic accuracy of this new technology, CCTA using 16-slice multidetector computed tomography (MDCT), against the reference or "gold" standard of ICA (see Figure 6.1). We were able to publish a relatively small study in the top *Cardiology Journal* [3]. In this section we provide practical advice on how we developed this study.

6.3.1 Costs/Budget

The planned time frame for this study was 1 year, allowing for roughly one patient per week, which is high (average NIH study enrolls one patient per month). The total budget was approximately $200K, which paid for a **clinical research coordinator (CRC)** to help with recruitment, CCTA and quantitative ICA reading workstations, data storage, the effort of the investigators, and the cost of the CCTAs.

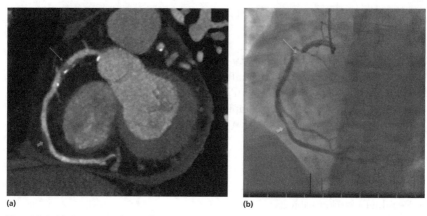

(a)   (b)

Figure 6.1 **(a)** Contrast enhanced coronary CT angiography (left) with severe stenosis of the right coronary artery (dark arrow) confirmed on **(b)** corresponding invasive catheter angiography (right).

6.3.2 Team

Even a small prospective trial requires a team approach. In this case the team consisted of the PI, a cardiologist to provide the clinical perspective, an interventional cardiologist to perform the blinded ICA reads and recruit the patients, at least two readers for CT so that interreader variability can be assessed, a statistician to perform the statistical analysis, and a support team consisting of a CRC to assist with patient recruitment, case report from (CRF) documentation, data management and anonymization, assistance with IRB issues, and other administrative work.

6.3.3 Feasibility

In order to convince your colleagues, let alone a funding agency, to support your trial, you must answer a series of critical, practical questions about feasibility. First, do you have a sufficient pool of patients to recruit into your trial? For this study, through our invasive cardiology colleagues, we knew that our site did approximately 3000 ICAs per year. Second, will the outcome (significant coronary stenosis) be common enough to see an effect in your population sample? We knew that about half of the ICAs performed at our facility had known CAD. By limiting our inclusion criteria to those with known CAD, we enriched the frequency of the outcome to ensure that we would have a reasonable chance at assessing accuracy (see Chapter 7 for more on enrichment and other design strategies to increase study power). Third, is the trial ethical? As in drug trials, there must be a state of equipoise (see Chapter 7). Any trial exposes subjects to tests or dangers that they would not otherwise face, in this case the risk of contrast nephropathy, radiation exposure, and potentially delay to care. You must design the study to minimize these risks to the subjects. Fourth, you must have a good working relationship with your colleagues who will be referring your subjects.

6.3.4 Good practices

Choose a good imaging acquisition protocol and stick to it. The natural tendency is towards drift—changes in protocol with evolution in your clinical protocols, such as a new imaging equipment vendor. In most cases it is best to resist change and stick with the protocol once the study is underway. Data collection and quality control should be a continuous process. It is easy to fall into the trap of focusing all of your energy on patient recruitment and the day-to-day tasks of running the study. Be sure to also perform quality control as the data comes in so you can anticipate problems and, if necessary, get further follow-up. It is a difficult but common situation to be a year or more into a trial and then realize that a key data element is missing for a substantial number of subjects—practice continuous quality assurance of your data as it comes in to avoid this. Bias can be partially avoided with blinded data interpretation (see Chapter 7 for descriptions of various biases common in imaging trials). Imaging studies should be deidentified, and readers should be blinded to the clinical scenario and results of other tests. When possible, having multiple observers will allow you to quantify interobserver variability, a must with any new imaging test.

6.3.5 Multicenter trials

This study was the first US experience published with the new technology. The data helped to get larger studies funded by NIH and others. Challenges/opportunities from running a multicenter trial are somewhat different and include site selection, contracts, incentivization, multicenter IRBs, organization of a multicenter study team, committees and delegation, multisite level randomization, central data repository, electronic data management systems, independent adjudication of clinical events, and data safety monitoring boards (DSMBs). Multicenter trials usually are quite expensive ($20–70 million) and usually require forming several cores: Imaging core, Biomarker core, Outcomes core, Statistical core, Data Management core, Budget and Contracting core, and IRB core.

6.4 Operational aspects of conducting a clinical trial

The second part of this chapter outlines the practicalities of running a trial from a more operational perspective. The main components to consider when organizing a trial include:
- Investigator team and environment
- Standard operating procedures
- Federal and local research compliance
- Pre- and post-award

6.4.1 Good clinical practice (GCP)

The principle of conducting a clinical trial is led by "good clinical practice" (GCP). GCP applies to all aspects of clinical trial conduct including monitoring, enrollment, auditing, reporting, data management, and analysis. Guidelines are maintained on the website of the International Conference on Harmonization of Technical Requirements for Registration of Pharmaceuticals for Human Use (ICH) that governs the responsibilities of investigators, sponsors, and monitors involved in clinical studies to ensure the quality and integrity of the study data.

6.4.2 The principal investigator

The investigator is responsible for the oversight and ultimate success of the trial but needs an experienced team to ensure a structured working environment and a smooth trial. Table 6.3 summarizes important obligations for PIs.

The novice investigator should recognize the need to clearly outline all trial activities. This is best accomplished through a set of **standard operating procedures (SOPs)**. SOPs provide stability and consistency throughout a trial. They are central to any trial and serve as a framework and resource for team members for the trial operations to ensure consistency. A comprehensive set of SOPs should cover all trial activities, including site initiation and study start-up, imaging protocol, data management, quality assurance, and reviewer training and conduct. An example of a basic SOP library for an imaging study is shown in Figure 6.2.

For large clinical trials an imaging core lab is required but the following elements are important for any study collecting and storing image data sets or conducting reads.

6.4.3 Data security

Data sharing and security are important issues and relevant for non-imaging and imaging data elements. As such, all institutional SOPs apply to clinical trial operations. Additionally, clinical trials may use equipment reserved exclusively for

Table 6.3 Obligations for PIs.

Pay attention to adverse events	Promptly document deviations from protocol, premature unbinding, adverse events not covered by protocol, etc.
Pay attention to informed consent documents	IRB approval of every revision
	Language should be understandable and as nontechnical as possible
	List of required disclosures included in guidelines
Ensure accuracy, completeness, legibility, and timeliness of data	Do not backdate
	Use only blue or black ink on paper source documents
Retain records for 2 years	Local regulations may dictate longer retention period; check with your institution

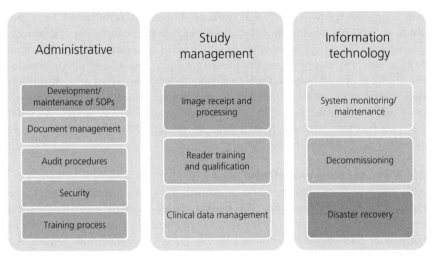

Figure 6.2 Components of an SOP for an imaging trial.

clinical and/or imaging trials and therefore an established library of SOPs, covering procedures and controls tailored to the conduct required for imaging clinical trials, and ensuring full compliance with federal and local regulations needs to be maintained. These SOPs should pertain to user accounts and security, facilities, network security, account management, clinical trial data management system, central database, electronic document data storage, secure file transfer, and imaging systems including Quality Assurance/Quality Control (QA/QC) Workstations and PACS/RIS.

6.4.4 Study management

Study management is a complex operation that starts with site selection, training, and certification and extends to all site documents including manual of operations, study protocol, and clinical report forms. From an operational point of view, it includes contracting sites, IRB approval of sites, interactions with the DSMB, sponsor, and adjudication of events. It is very important to form relationships with your sites so they will follow instructions. This can be achieved by taking the time to train at the start of the study and ensuring you have an adequate number of clinical research associates (CRAs) for monitoring. Also make contacts with the right people for imaging (lead imaging physicians and technologists) and ensure that they are in fact seen as part of the trial team.

SOPs are important to build consistency across trials and constitute a source of knowledge and help with any trial. An SOP repository should be built to help mastering the operational and regulatory challenges. Template SOPs create uniformity in the performance of a specific function. In the instance of new or inexperienced research staff, SOPs are an important resource as standard, study-specific documentation that should enable them to follow the process consistently. For IT SOPs documenting the use of computer systems, it is vital to eliminate any errors, especially those that could result in errors or delay of the tracking of trial information. Common technical systems and procedures that should undergo testing include secure storage location/file system (hard-copy and electronic docs), electronic imaging data transfer system (secure, encrypted), image archival system (e.g., an internal PACS), and data capture system (e.g., eCRF programming).

6.4.5 Processing workflow

After these systems are tested and confirmed, a processing workflow SOP (see Figure 6.3) should be developed. This workflow functions to ensure data collected are received from the site; once the data are received, they become the responsibility of the trial operations team to perform quality assurance. For example, the trial CRAs receive a data set with patient information on the images. There must be predetermined procedures for these situations. They must have procedures/ tools in place to adequately scrub private health information (PHI) and to train sites to anonymize images prior to submission—if they do not adhere, send a query requiring their response rather than a reminder.

The typical standard study documentation includes the following SOPs:
- Project Plan
- Communication Plan
- Core Lab Manual
- Reviewer Training Manual/Review Charter
- Image Acquisition Guidelines (IAGs)
- Image Submission Guidelines (ISGs)
- Image Record Forms (IRFs)

The CRA should follow a standard workflow for the QA/QC process. In the instance of image receipt, the process should include image protocol checks (did the site adhere?), correct anatomical coverage, radiation dose monitoring, if applicable, checks for proper anonymization, tracking and archival, and, if possible, a second CRA to perform a second QC (industry sponsors sometimes require this).

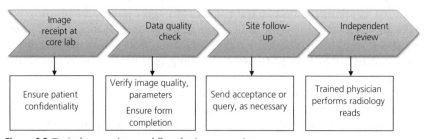

Figure 6.3 Typical processing workflow for image receipts.

6.5 Audits

In addition to an awareness of GCP, in the case of an industry trial, audits are a common practice. Industry sponsors request an audit of SOPs and facilities at least once over the course of each project. This often occurs at the start of the project.

In a typical audit for an industry-sponsored study, they will often request an audit of your facilities to review your SOPs (Are they up to date? Did you perform all internal audits as scheduled? Is everyone's training documented?) and to ensure all systems are in compliance with your SOPs and GCPs (e.g., PSs auto lock after 5 min and areas of restricted access are maintained, documentation from other sponsors is not out in the open). You should request an agenda and a listing of documents they wish to see in advance—have photocopies prepared and do not provide originals. Follow your own rules. If you have an audit SOP (and you should), make sure you follow the procedures therein.

In addition to sponsor audits, the FDA may audit you without notice. A **surveillance inspection** is a routine general inspection that usually focuses on basic FDA regulations and GCP compliance. A **compliance inspection** may arise in response to one of two scenarios: (i) A suspected violation of FDA regulations (also called **for-cause**) or (ii) a drug seeking FDA approval has prompted a review by sponsor, manufacturer, or FDA because of suspected unsafe data or procedures. You should obtain a copy of the inspection report from the Freedom of Information Office after 30 days from the audit. Some observations require a formal response; provide written response within 30 business days of inspection conclusion.

The operational success of a clinical trial orbits around the need for well-developed SOPs. Once these are in place, nearly any issue can be resolved by referring to procedure. From the training of study personnel to the tracking and processing of all data, these processes can all be referenced in the SOP.

6.6 Summary

Engaging in clinical research and trials is not practical but can be very exciting. Some of the prerequisites for success we have outlined in this chapter are (i) highly significant topic with potential to feed a research career rather than a single study, (ii) smart choice of type of study guided by a match of the complexity with investigators' experience and the institutional environment, (iii) help from a mentor that can maneuver you through hurdles with institutional support, team building, and funding, (iv) organization of trial documents, (v) meticulous planning for all aspects of a trial ahead of time, and finally (vi) leadership—have conviction and enthusiasm and create a team.

References

1 Gazelle, G.S., et al., A framework for assessing the value of diagnostic imaging in the era of comparative effectiveness research. *Radiology*, 2011. **261**(3): p. 692–698.

2 Franklin, B., Advice to a Young Tradesman, Written by an Old One. 1748; Available from: http://ebooks.cambridge.org/chapter.jsf?bid=CBO9780511806889&cid=CBO978051180688 9A027).

3 Hoffmann, U., et al., Predictive value of 16-slice multidetector spiral computed tomography to detect significant obstructive coronary artery disease in patients at high risk for coronary artery disease: patient-versus segment-based analysis. *Circulation*, 2004. **110**(17): p. 2638–2643.

CHAPTER 7

Statistical issues in study design

Nancy A. Obuchowski

Quantitative Health Sciences, Cleveland Clinic Foundation, Cleveland, OH, USA

KEY POINTS

- The common building blocks of imaging studies include a detailed research question, a description of the imaging test(s), a valid reference standard, representative study samples (both subjects and readers), and sensitive and meaningful study endpoints.

- "Accuracy" is a stronger measure of a modality's performance than either "agreement" or "correlation." Studies of diagnostic accuracy require a reference standard.

- Verification bias is one of the most common biases in imaging studies, often falsely inflating estimates of sensitivity and underestimating specificity. It occurs when the test results influence decisions about which subjects undergo the reference standard.

- Sample size calculations are a vital part of study design and should take into account the primary study objective, the study design, and conservative assumptions about the unknown data.

7.1 Diversity in imaging study designs

In the first six chapters, we heard about a variety of imaging studies and their design, phases of the technologies' assessment, and a range of research questions. In this chapter we discuss the building blocks of an imaging research study, common biases in these studies, strategies for efficient designs, and sample size considerations. Throughout the chapter we illustrate study design ideas using the case examples from Chapter 1.

7.2 Building blocks of an imaging research study

Imaging studies typically have five common building blocks: a research question, study sample (subjects and sometimes readers), imaging test, reference standard (if applicable), and study outcomes:

Handbook for Clinical Trials of Imaging and Image-Guided Interventions, First Edition.
Edited by Nancy A. Obuchowski and G. Scott Gazelle.
© 2016 John Wiley & Sons, Inc. Published 2016 by John Wiley & Sons, Inc.

- The **research question** should be consistent with the technological assessment phase of the modality, as discussed in Chapter 1. This requires a thorough literature review to allow investigators to determine which research questions have already been addressed and what are the next logical questions to be asked.
- The **imaging test** includes the technical parameters of the modality under investigation, how and by whom it will be interpreted, and a description of any competing tests.
- The **reference standard** is required in studies assessing diagnostic test accuracy. The choice of a reference standard depends on the phase of the technical assessment and the goals of the study. We discuss this further in Section 7.2.3.
- The **study sample** includes not only a description of the characteristics of the sample of subjects to be studied but also the readers who interpret the tests or perform the interventions. See Section 7.2.2 for further details.
- The **study endpoints** (or outcomes) are the quantitative and/or qualitative measurements determined for each study subject. Studies typically have a primary endpoint and one or more secondary endpoints. Often these endpoints coincide with the primary and secondary objectives of the study. Sample size assessments are usually performed for the primary endpoint only. In imaging studies the endpoints range from technical performance (e.g., measurement bias, repeatability, reproducibility; see Chapter 10), diagnostic accuracy (e.g., ROC analyses; see Chapter 9), patient outcomes (e.g., time until recurrence), and finally societal outcomes (e.g., cost-effectiveness; see Chapter 11). Figure 7.1 illustrates the building blocks for Case example 1.2.

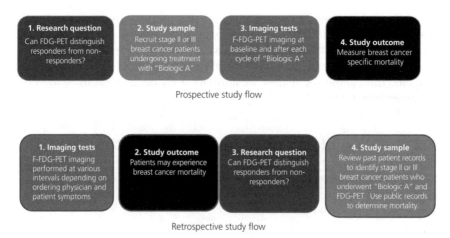

Figure 7.1 Building blocks of imaging studies. The figure illustrates the typical workflow for prospective and retrospective designs for Case example 1.2. Note that for this study there is no reference standard.

7.2.1 Turning research questions into study objectives and statistical hypotheses

There are two types of research questions: pragmatic and explanatory [1]. A **pragmatic** research question asks whether an imaging modality works under real-life conditions and whether it helps in the diagnosis and/or management of patients; it does not delve into the biology or imaging technology to address why it works. An **explanatory** research question, however, asks why and how the modality works. For a pragmatic research question, we would typically want a sample of patients and readers representative of their respective population so that our study results will be generalizable to these populations. On the other hand, in an explanatory study we might want to focus on a homogeneous group of patients (or even phantoms) to try to understand how and why the imaging test works or fails to work. Of course, sometimes studies include both types of questions.

Regardless of the type of research question, a critical step in designing a study is turning the research question into a study objective, from which the statistical analysis plan can be formulated. A **study objective** is an active statement about the specific steps you will take to answer the research question. The study objective formalizes the research question to state very specifically how and what will be evaluated and by whom. The objective should not state the research hypothesis, and it should not include any language about the investigators' hope for a statistically significant finding. Rather, it should be an objective statement about how and what will be tested or measured. Figure 7.2 illustrates the process for

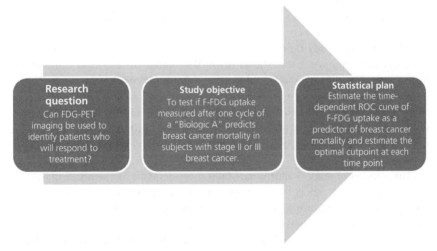

Figure 7.2 Turning research question to statistical plan. Case example 1.2 is used to illustrate a typical research question, study objective, and brief statistical plan.

Case example 1.2. The study objective should include the independent variables (e.g., ^{18}F-FDP update) and outcome variables (breast cancer mortality), the imaging modality being evaluated (^{18}F-FDG PET), and the clinical setting being studied (e.g., stage II and III breast cancer patients).

Once the study objective is formulated, the statistical analysis plan can be developed. The statistical analysis plan involves estimating unknown parameters and often testing a hypothesis about them. In Case example 1.2 we want to determine if ^{18}F-FDP update after treatment with "Biologic A" predicts breast cancer mortality. We discuss more about statistical hypotheses in Section 7.5.2.

7.2.2 Sampling from patient and reader populations

Guided by their research questions, investigators have a variety of options when sampling subjects and readers for retrospective and prospective designs. For some studies, investigators may need a homogeneous group of subjects (e.g., in a study of breast cancer, postmenopausal women with dense breasts) or a broad spectrum of subjects (e.g., all women presenting for screening). The advantage of the former is that there is less noise (i.e., variability) in the study, so often we can identify trends/associations easier. This is important in explanatory studies. The disadvantage is that the study results are applicable to a narrow subset of the population and we have no data on how well the test will perform for other subjects in the population. This would be problematic for a pragmatic study.

In imaging studies we often recruit subjects who are referred for imaging, overlooking other subjects who might meet our eligibility criteria but who were not referred for the imaging test. Referral patterns can distort the composition of our study samples; this can occur in both retrospective and prospective designs. We discuss spectrum bias in Section 7.4.1.

When we are studying modalities that require trained readers to interpret, it's important that we assess the effect of the reader on our study outcomes. Single reader studies are inadequate because the study results are specific to the lone reader in the study. Often investigators recruit readers exclusively from their home institution. If the readers have been trained at the same site, they will often perform similarly, whereas readers from different sites, or at least trained at different sites, may be more representative of the population of readers.

The number of readers appropriate for a study depends on the phase of the test assessment (fewer readers for early assessments of a new modality, more readers for assessments of mature modalities) and on the variability between the readers (the more variability between the readers, the more readers needed). In Section 7.5.4 we discuss sample size considerations for a **multireader multicase** (**MRMC**) study using Case example 1.1 for illustration. See Chapter 9 for discussion of the statistical analysis of MRMC studies.

7.2.3 What is a reference standard?

Zhou et al. [2] define a reference standard (they refer to it as a "gold standard") as "a source of information, completely different from the test or tests under evaluation, which tells us the true condition of the patient." This definition is more specific to diagnostic accuracy studies where the goal is to estimate test sensitivity and specificity. For diagnostic accuracy studies, reasonable reference standards include autopsy reports, surgery findings, pathology results, and findings from an invasive procedure. Sometimes more than one reference standard is needed in the same study. An example is a study of the accuracy of new modalities to screen for breast cancer. Subjects with positive test results might undergo additional testing including biopsy. Subjects who do not undergo biopsy might be followed with additional imaging at 1 year; if the 1-year images do not show cancer, then we can assume that the earlier images were free of cancer. Thus, both pathology and 1-year follow-up are reference standards for this type of study.

The term "reference standard" can also refer to a clinically acceptable test, or state-of-the-art method for diagnosing a condition. It may be imperfect as a source of information for estimating test accuracy but still considered the reference standard. We might be interested in determining how frequently a new test agrees with the reference standard; when the tests disagree, we cannot be certain which one is correct.

In studies with phantoms or digital reference images, we often have the "true value" (sometimes referred to as "ground truth"). For example, in a phantom study of pulmonary nodules, we know the true volume of the synthetic nodule in the image; thus, we can compare measurements made on the images to this true value.

Understanding the limitations of the reference standard is critical to determining how it can be used in the study. Sometimes in the early assessment of a new imaging modality, we are willing to use an imperfect reference standard to estimate the accuracy of the new test because if the new test shows good accuracy, then it will be evaluated in future studies, hopefully with a better reference standard. For mature modalities, nearly perfect reference standards are needed to properly estimate test accuracy. Sometimes investigators, in an effort to ensure that all subjects in the study have the proper reference standard, inadvertently introduce verification bias into their studies. We discuss this problem further in Section 7.4.2. When no reference standard is available, other strategies must be considered. One option is the formation of a panel of experts (i.e., "gold standard panel") who have all test results, history, and follow-up information on subjects from which to determine the "true" diagnosis (see Ref. [3]). This might be a reasonable approach for Case example 1.1, where a panel of experts might review all available clinical data within the last six months, including other imaging tests and biopsies. Another option is to forgo estimates of test accuracy and report how the test results affect patient outcome through patient decision-making [4, 5].

7.3 Strategies for efficient studies

In this section we discuss a variety of strategies for unbiased and/or efficient designs. Not all of them are applicable for each study.

7.3.1 Retrospective or prospective?

Both retrospective and prospective designs are common in imaging studies. In a retrospective study investigators collect data from past imaging records and clinical records; there is no new follow-up of subjects. The advantages of a retrospective study are (i) smaller sample sizes, (ii) shorter studies, and (iii) efficiency when studying rare conditions. The disadvantages of this design are introduction of bias, such as selection and verification bias (see Section 7.4), and lack of uniformity in the research procedures (i.e., varied imaging parameters and image interpretation and nonuniform subject assessment regarding specific outcomes and timing).

In a prospective study subjects are followed over time through the planned imaging test(s) and until the study outcome has been observed. A distinguishing feature of a prospective study is that at the time the investigators recruit subjects for the study, none of the subjects has developed any of the outcomes being tested. Prospective studies are typically ranked higher in the hierarchy of evidence than retrospective studies because there are usually fewer biases in a prospective design.

Some research questions can be addressed by either a prospective or retrospective design, while others are naturally suited to one type of design. Many diagnostic accuracy studies, like Case example 1.1, can be conducted retrospectively or prospectively. Usually the sample size is much smaller with a retrospective design because investigators can select the optimal number of subjects with and without the abnormality of interest, whereas at the start of a prospective design, investigators are uncertain about how many subjects with and without the condition will eventually be recruited. When a new modality is being evaluated, for example, a new ultrasound device for diagnosing breast lesions, a prospective design may be required if the new device has not been used yet in clinical practice. In Case examples 1.2 and 1.3, a review of past clinical data might aid investigators in determining the optimal imaging parameters and provide a rough idea of the expected outcomes. A prospective design for Case example 1.2, however, would provide a more valid assessment of the prediction ability of ^{18}F-FDG uptake because the imaging can be performed at uniform times and with a uniform procedure. Also, probability models of breast cancer mortality can be constructed from a representative sample of breast cancer subjects, rather than a potentially biased sample of subjects who happened to undergo FDG PET. Figure 7.1 compares the workflow of a prospective and retrospective design for this example, illustrating the problems associated with a retrospective review to find study subjects. Similarly, an equitable comparison of minimally invasive therapies

(Case example 1.3) can be performed only in a prospective design by randomizing subjects, rather than relying on statistical modeling to try to account for differences in sample compositions of historical patients.

7.3.2 Paired designs

Many imaging studies use paired designs for their efficiency. In a **paired design** each study subject undergoes the two or more modalities under evaluation. For example, in Case example 1.1 each subject might be imaged with Agents A and B on different days. Alternatively, in an **unpaired design** one sample of subjects would be imaged with Agent A and a different sample of subjects would be imaged with Agent B. The main advantages of a paired design over an unpaired design are a smaller sample size (by reducing the variability) and control over potentially confounding variables. In fact, paired designs control for confounding variables even better than randomization. Randomization results in similar subject and disease characteristics in the study arms *over the long run* (i.e., after a large number of subjects are randomized); paired designs guarantee the same subject and disease characteristics for any sample size. One potential disadvantage of a paired design is an ordering effect whereby one modality has an advantage because it is always performed first (or last). For example, in a diagnostic accuracy study, one modality might have an advantage if it is always performed in closer proximity in time to the reference standard. Ordering effects can be eliminated by randomizing the order in which the modalities are performed.

When the modalities are mutually exclusive (e.g., due to their invasiveness or expense) or when the study outcome cannot be evaluated specific to the imaging, a paired design cannot be used. In Case example 1.3 one group of subjects would undergo RFA and a different sample of subjects would undergo SABR; the therapies are mutually exclusive, so pairing is not possible. Furthermore, the study outcome is progression-free survival, which does not lend itself to a paired design.

In MRMC studies, designs can include subjects and readers both paired, both unpaired, or any combination. In a paired reader, paired subject design, subjects undergo all imaging tests being evaluated, and then readers interpret the images from both tests. In an unpaired reader, unpaired subject design, different subjects undergo the imaging tests and different readers interpret the images from each test. Unpaired reader designs are uncommon in imaging studies but would be required if readers were unable, due to lack of training or experience, to interpret the images from both tests. In Section 7.5.4 we will discuss the differences in sample size requirements for paired and unpaired MRMC designs.

7.3.3 Augmented and enriched designs

In diagnostic accuracy studies when the natural prevalence of disease is low, investigators often augment the study sample to increase the study prevalence. For example, in Case example 1.1 if we were to use a retrospective design, we might select a higher frequency of subjects who are known to have liver metastases than we might observe by simply selecting consecutive eligible subjects.

This is one of the important advantages of a retrospective design (see Section 7.5.4 for illustration of the effect on sample size requirements). In a prospective design we can augment the prevalence in the study sample by using stratified or two-stage sampling. In stratified sampling we first group subjects based on characteristics known to be associated with the disease. Then we optimally recruit subjects from these groups (i.e., strata), oversampling from the groups with the highest prevalence rates. In the second strategy, all subjects first undergo the diagnostic test (stage I). Then we sample subjects to undergo the reference standard (stage II) based on their results from the first phase, oversampling the subjects with a positive test result. As long as we randomly sample subjects based on the results from the first stage, and we know the sampling rates that we applied, then in the analysis we can adjust study outcomes for the type and rate of sampling [6].

A different concept is enrichment whereby investigators include subjects with particular characteristics in order to evaluate the performance of the imaging modality for these subjects. In Case example 1.2 we might recruit a predetermined number of subjects with stage II and stage III breast cancers because we want to ensure that we have enough statistical power to test the predictive ability of FDP-PET for both of these important patient groups. Alternatively, if we were to recruit consecutive subjects, we might have too few stage III subjects to evaluate study outcome on these patients.

7.3.4 Randomization

Randomization is used in imaging studies to generate comparable groups prior to comparing interventions or to comparing modalities' accuracies when a paired design cannot be used. In Case example 1.3 randomization should be used to generate two comparable groups where subjects in each group undergo one of the two invasive procedures. In Case example 1.1 the two blood-pool agents cannot be easily performed on the same subjects, so subjects could be randomized to one of the two agents. Randomization is also used to generate the order of the lists of images for study readers to interpret; this prevents readers from remembering cases and ensures that images of all one type are not read last when readers might be more fatigued or more accustomed to the evaluations.

Randomization can only be used when there is equipoise. The *principle of equipoise* provides the ethical basis for the use of randomization in a clinical trial. **Equipoise** "occurs if there is genuine uncertainty within the expert medical community—not necessarily on the part of the individual investigator—about the preferred treatment" [7].

There are different procedures for randomizing subjects. In **simple randomization**, there is a single sequence of random assignments from which subjects are assigned to the different groups. A computer-generated randomization list can be created in the design phase of a study from which numbered sealed envelopes are generated containing the study assignment for each subject. Study investigators use the envelopes, in order, to determine each new subject's assignment. The disadvantage of simple randomization is that in small studies the number of subjects in each study arm can be imbalanced. **Block randomization** overcomes the imbalance problem. Randomization is performed in small blocks, so that at the end of each block, there is balance between the arms of the study. A disadvantage of both simple and block randomization is that, particularly in small studies, there can be imbalances in subject covariates (i.e., for a study of breast cancer, there could be more subjects with palpable lesions in one arm than the other). **Stratified randomization** can be used to ensure balance between study arms for baseline covariates known to be related to the study outcome. Stratified randomization is achieved by generating separate blocks for each combination of covariates. A subject's covariates are evaluated at baseline and then the subject is assigned to the corresponding stratum from which she or he is randomized.

Consider the randomization scheme for Case example 1.3. We may want to stratify subjects based on the stage of lung cancer, age, and comorbidities because we feel that these variables strongly affect our study outcome, progression-free survival. If we group stage I with II and III with IV, patient age into less than 60 and greater than or equal to 60 years, and comorbidities into presence/absence of COPD, then we would have 2 stages × 2 ages × 2 comorbidities = 8 randomization strata. Within each of these strata, we may want to create blocks of, say, 4, so that for every four subjects enrolled with this particular configuration of covariates, two will undergo RFA and two will undergo SABR. This stratified, block randomization scheme is quite complicated to set up and implement. Investigators would need to weigh the complexities against the benefits during the design phase of the study.

Randomization is not a straightforward ticket to an unbiased or efficient study, especially in imaging. Imaging studies provide information that affect patient decision-making by influencing the ordering of other diagnostic tests and determining the best treatment plan. These events have a large impact on patient outcomes. Consider an RCT where subjects are randomized to modality A or B. Depending on the test results, subjects undergo different treatment and then patient outcome (e.g., survival) is assessed. The study is thus a comparison of the effect of both the diagnostic test *and treatment* on patient outcome; it is not solely a comparison of the effect of the diagnostic test on patient outcome, which may have been the goal of the study. Bossuyt et al. [8], Lijmer and Bossuyt [5], and Lu and Gatsonis [9] discuss the limitations of RCTs in evaluating the effect of diagnostic tests on patient outcome and describe some alternatives. One alternative is depicted in Figure 7.3 where subjects undergo both modalities A and B, and only subjects where the test results of A and B disagree are randomized.

7.3.5 Interim analyses

In prospective studies investigators often want to assess the study findings before the end of the trial. For example, investigators may want to evaluate the safety of a new modality before too many subjects are enrolled. They may also want to

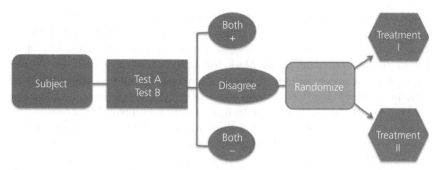

Figure 7.3 RCT to assess effect of imaging on patient outcome. Instead of randomizing subjects to undergo either test A or B, subjects undergo both tests A and B, and then those with discordant results are randomized.

determine if the study should be terminated early because the results are unimpressive (futility) or very impressive (benefit). These so-called **interim analyses** must be planned in the design phase of the study.

There are a variety of methods for planning interim analyses. These methods account for the fact that the investigators are performing multiple analyses of the data instead of just one analysis at the end of the study. Each time investigators test the study hypotheses, they risk a type I error. For example, suppose the study's null hypothesis is that F-FDG update does not predict breast cancer mortality, while the alternative hypothesis is that F-FDG update does predict breast cancer mortality. A type I error occurs when F-FDG update is truly not associated with mortality, yet the p-value for the test statistic is small enough so that we reject the null hypothesis. Over the course of a study, the test statistic, which is used to test the study hypotheses, randomly fluctuates in magnitude. The more often investigators test the study hypotheses, the greater the risk that at some testing point, the test statistic will be falsely high, leading to a type I error.

Investigators set up **stopping rules** to control the study's overall type I error rate at a specified level (using 5%). Two commonly used stopping rule methods are the Pocock method and the O'Brien–Fleming method [10, 11]. These two methods "spend" the study's overall type I error rate in different ways. Suppose that investigators decide that they will perform two interim analyses after one-third and two-thirds of the data are collected and then a final study analysis after all study subjects are enrolled. According to the Pocock method, for each of the three analyses, a significance level of 0.022 is used to evaluate the study's p-values. In contrast, with the O'Brien–Fleming method, a significance level of 0.0005 is used for the first analysis, 0.014 for the second analysis, and 0.045 for the final analysis. Both methods, however, result in an overall study type I error rate of 0.05 (5%).

For further details on stopping rules and adaptive study designs, readers are encouraged to consult Barker et al. [12], Chin [13], Chow and Chang [14], Jennison and Turnbull [15], and Whitehead [16].

7.4 Common biases in imaging studies

The word "bias" means a systematic error that occurs sometimes when designing a study (i.e., **design bias**) and sometimes when we are making measurements (we will discuss **measurement bias** in Chapter 10). Note that systematic error differs from random error, in that systematic errors are reproducible errors that occur consistently in the same direction, whereas random errors are unpredictable. Random error will be discussed in Chapter 8.

Investigators want to minimize design bias because they care about the validity of their study, that is, we want to be sure that we get a truthful result from our study. For example, in a study of the relative accuracy of two modalities showing that modality A is more accurate than modality B, we want to be assured that this result is truthful, even if it is truthful only for the patients and readers involved in our study. This is akin to **internal validity** [17]. A type of bias common in the imaging literature that can compromise this validity is verification bias (see Section 7.4.2). Taking this a step further, **external validity** means that the study results are generalizable to other institutions, that is, modality A is more accurate than modality B at other institutions. Spectrum bias (Section 7.4.1) is an example of a bias that can compromise external validity.

Design biases are common in research studies. Their effects vary depending on the type and magnitude of the bias. Investigators often design studies, recognizing that bias exists in the design they have chosen but realizing there is no practical alternative to avoid the bias. In these situations investigators need to be sure that the effect of the bias won't compromise the internal validity. Table 7.1 summarizes several types of design biases in imaging studies and the nature of their threat to the study's validity. Strategies to minimize the effects of the bias are presented, classified as A, B, or C according to whether the strategy avoids, minimizes, or adjusts for the bias, respectively.

We focus now on two important biases (i.e., spectrum and verification bias).

7.4.1 Spectrum bias

Spectrum bias occurs when the outcome of the imaging test you are studying depends on characteristics of the study sample and your study sample is not representative of the relevant population. For example, suppose you are studying the accuracy of breast tomosynthesis for detecting cancer. Its sensitivity is likely positively correlated with lesion size. If your study sample was composed exclusively of women with palpable lesions, then spectrum bias exists because your estimate of sensitivity will be too high (i.e., higher than the true sensitivity when calculated from all women presenting for breast screening).

To avoid spectrum bias, investigators need to consider disease characteristics (e.g., lesion sizes, location of abnormality), patient characteristics (e.g., breast densities, patients' age), imaging device characteristics (e.g., manufacturer), and

Table 7.1 Common biases in imaging studies.

Bias	Description	Threat	Strategies to minimize bias*
Spectrum	Subject or reader sample does not include full spectrum of subject/reader characteristics that affect study outcome	External validity	Identify key characteristics and recruit representative subjects/readers (A). Estimate and report study outcomes by key characteristics (B).
Referral	Only subjects referred for imaging compose the study sample, altering the true relative frequencies of subgroups	External validity	Collaborate with PCPs to recruit patients for better representation (A).
Verification	Test results affect which patients undergo reference standard and only subjects undergoing reference standard are included in study	Internal validity	Design study so that test results don't influence decisions about reference standard (A). Include multiple reference standards (B). Model the bias (C).
Imperfect reference standard	Reference standard does not provide true diagnosis of subject, leading to biased estimates of test accuracy.	Internal validity	Identify a better reference standard for study (A). Model the bias (C).
Incorporation	Bias typically occurs when reference standard is a compilation of findings from various tests and/or patient outcome. Bias is when reference standard is based in part on results of test(s) under study.	Internal validity	Ensure that reference standard is independent of test(s) under study (A).
Disease progression	Disease progresses between time when test and reference standard are performed	Internal validity	Shorten interval between test and reference standard (B). Statistical modeling can assess magnitude of bias (C).
Review	Test and/or reference standard are performed without proper blinding of readers	Internal validity	Mask readers to reference standard results when performing and interpreting test, and vice versa (A)
Reading order	Readers' recall of images or their increasing experience with interpreting a type of image lead to an advantage	Internal validity	Randomize reading order of images so that ordering doesn't favor one test (B)
Location	Readers get credit for correctly identifying subjects with an abnormality even when they mislocate the lesion.	Internal validity	Require readers to correctly locate lesion to get credit for correct diagnosis (A).

*A, strategies avoid the bias; B, strategies minimize the bias; and C, strategies adjust study results for the bias.

reader characteristics (e.g., board-certified mammographers of different experience levels, imagers working under different practice models) that might affect the outcome of the study. If it's impractical to include a broad spectrum of subjects and/or readers, investigators should recognize and state the relevant patient and reader populations that the study findings represent. Investigators should also report how subject and reader characteristics affect the study outcome (e.g., report sensitivity for different lesion sizes and for readers of different experience levels). This allows investigators at other sites, where subjects' and readers' characteristics may differ, to assess how the test will perform at their institution.

Consider an example where efforts were made to avoid spectrum bias. Jarvik et al. [18] studied patients with low back pain whose physician ordered a radiograph. The investigators randomized patients to either rapid MRI or plain film and then followed them to assess their functional status. Note that the authors clearly described their patient population, generalizing the study findings to patients with low back pain, not necessarily to all patients undergoing lumbar spine radiographs. The investigators recruited patients from four geographically diverse sites (two private centers, one university-based center, and one nonuniversity teaching center). The recruitment from multiple sites was performed to include a broad spectrum of patients, imagers, and device characteristics (i.e., avoiding spectrum bias and providing external validity).

7.4.2 Verification bias

Verification bias occurs in diagnostic accuracy studies when the test results of the modality under investigation are compared (*verified*) with the results of the reference standard but not all study subjects undergo the reference standard. In clinical practice the test results from the modality under investigation sometimes influence the decision of whether or not to perform the reference standard. When this occurs and subjects are excluded from a diagnostic accuracy study because they did not undergo the reference standard, verification bias has occurred. Figure 7.4 illustrates the problem. Subjects with negative test results, which include both true negatives and false negatives, tend not to undergo the reference standard, especially if the reference standard is invasive, costly, or time-consuming. When subjects with negative test results are excluded from the study, even if it is just a small subset of the study sample, estimates of test accuracy will be skewed. Usually sensitivity is overestimated (because some of the false negatives have been excluded from the study) and specificity is underestimated (because some of the true negatives have been excluded from the study). It is important to note that this bias occurs in both prospective and retrospective diagnostic accuracy studies and that increasing the overall sample size does not remove the bias.

Case example 1.1 is a diagnostic accuracy study prone to verification bias. Subjects who test negative for liver metastases would not typically undergo the reference standard. There are several possible strategies to avoid or minimize this bias. First, investigators can design the study such that all subjects would undergo

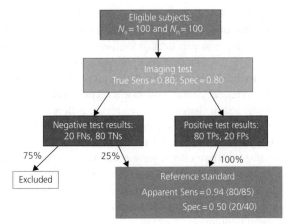

Figure 7.4 Illustration of effects of verification bias. Seventy-five percent of subjects with negative test results do not undergo the reference standard. The true sensitivity and specificity of the test is 0.80, but after verification bias the apparent sensitivity is 0.94 and the specificity is 0.50.

the reference standard regardless of their test results. Sometimes it is possible to recruit only subjects who are scheduled for the reference standard, consenting them to perhaps additional testing before or after the reference standard is performed. Sometimes it is feasible to blind subjects and investigators to the test results until the reference standard has been performed. A second strategy is multiple reference standards. For some abnormalities, there is more than one reference standard and sometimes it is clinically acceptable to perform one of multiple possible reference standards on all study subjects. There are also multiple statistical approaches to correcting estimates of accuracy for the presence of verification bias [2]. These approaches require investigators to collect data (i.e., test results and patient characteristics) on all subjects, regardless of whether or not they underwent the reference standard. This data is then used to correct estimates of accuracy for the bias.

7.5 Sample size considerations

Planning the size of a research study is a critical component of the study design phase. The sample size needed for a study can tell us if a study is feasible or not, how long the study will take, and what it will cost. We often refer to this part of the study design as **sample size considerations**, rather than sample size *determination*, because there are many unknowns in calculating the required sample. There are also resource limitations imposed on any study. All of these factors weigh into investigators' consideration of the appropriate sample size for the study.

7.5.1 Underpowered studies: clinical versus statistical significance

When the sample size is too small for meeting the goals of a study, we call the study "underpowered." The problem with underpowered studies is that they waste resources and they can mislead us.

Consider the study by Jarvik et al. [18] of rapid MRI for diagnosing back pain, which we discussed in Section 7.4.1. Jarvik et al. found no statistically significant difference (i.e., p-value >0.05) in the functional status scores of subjects in the two study arms. The mean scores were 8.75 (X-ray) and 9.34 (MRI) with a 95% CI for the difference of −1.69 to +0.87. What can the investigators conclude from this result? In the planning phase of the study, the authors made several critical decisions, which later affected what they could conclude from these results. First, they determined that a clinically important difference in functional scores was 2.0 or larger; a difference smaller than 2.0 was not important clinically. This is what is called the **clinically relevant difference**. Second, they planned for and carried out a study with a sample size large enough to detect a difference of 2.0 with a certain level of assuredness (i.e., statisticians call this the study's "power;" see Chapter 8 for a more detailed discussion of power, type I and II errors, and p-values). Lastly, concerned about possible dropouts from their study, they increased their initial sample size calculations by 15%.

Years after making these critical decisions, the investigators concluded that there is no difference in patients' functional status based on whether they underwent MRI or X-ray imaging. Their rationale was based on the fact that the p-value was not significant and the CI did not contain values greater than or equal to 2.0 or less than or equal to −2.0 (i.e., the CI was sufficiently narrow to rule out these values).

In contrast, consider their conclusions if the clinically relevant difference had instead been 1.0. They still would have found no statistically significant difference (i.e., p-value >0.05). Based on a p-value >0.05, a naïve investigator might immediately conclude that there is no difference; however, this would be misleading. Note that −1.0 is contained in the 95% CI; we cannot rule out the possibility that subjects who undergo MRI have clinically higher scores than those undergoing X-ray. The study would have been underpowered to detect a clinically relevant difference of 1.0. The investigators could neither conclude that the modalities have the same effect on functional status nor conclude that MRI leads to higher scores. The study would have been an expensive waste of resources.

7.5.2 Factors affecting sample size

The first step in sample size planning is determining the parameters that must be estimated and what we want to know or test about these parameters. For example, if the research question is simply what is the accuracy of a new modality, then the parameter we want to estimate might be the new modality's sensitivity and specificity, or its area under the ROC curve. If the research question is to compare the new modality with an existing modality (which we will refer to simply as the "old" modality), then we often want to test a hypothesis. The **null hypothesis** often expresses the commonly held belief about the parameter of interest, which the **alternative hypothesis** expresses a new conclusion. For example, the commonly held belief about a new modality is that its sensitivity is not as good as the old modality; this notion would be expressed in the null hypothesis. The researchers may believe that the new modality has superior sensitivity, so their belief would be expressed in the alternative hypothesis. (See Chapter 8 for different types of statistical hypotheses.)

The next step is often the most difficult: determining reasonable *guestimates* of the parameters of interest and their variability. It's ironic that the goal of the study is to estimate parameters, yet to plan the study we rely on approximations of these unknown parameters. We usually specify a likely range for the unknown parameters, and we often anchor the likely range by a conservative approximation of the parameters. For example, if the parameter of interest is the sensitivity of a new modality, and if there is no pilot data to get an approximation, then a conservative estimate is Sens = 0.5. Note that sensitivity is a proportion, that is, the proportion of abnormal subjects with a positive test result. Statistically, the variance of a proportion is $\text{Var}(p) = p \times (1-p)$. The maximum variance occurs when $p = 0.5$. Thus, setting Sens = 0.5 for sample size planning will lead to larger estimates of sample size (i.e., conservative estimate). Similarly, the variance of the AUC is related to the magnitude of the AUC, so choosing lower values for AUC in planning sample size will lead to conservative estimates of the sample size.

The third step really controls the sample size. If we are constructing a CI for our parameter, we must determine how narrow we want the CI to be. The more narrow the interval, the larger the required sample size. So deciding on how narrow the CI needs to be controls the sample size. When we are testing a hypothesis, we want some assuredness that we will reject the null hypothesis, in favor of the alternative hypothesis, when the alternative hypothesis is true. This is called the **power** of the study (see Chapter 8 for full discussion of the concept of power). The more power desired, the larger the required sample size. So deciding on the power controls the sample size.

Table 7.2 lists and defines these steps in planning sample size.

7.5.3 Sample size calculations

Most sample size calculations for imaging studies require an experienced statistician to perform. The reason is that most imaging studies are complicated. There are often multiple lesions in the same patient, and the correlation between lesions from the same patient must be accounted for in the sample size calculation. In prospective studies key factors of the sample size calculation are unknown (e.g., prevalence of abnormal patients in study sample), so the uncertainty in these factors must be taken into account. Time-to-event endpoints (e.g., time to recurrence) require assumptions about the pattern of patient accrual, pattern of

Table 7.2 Steps in sample size calculations.

Factors to consider	Interpretation
Step 1:	
What is the parameter of interest (we call it θ)?	The metric that you want to measure and compare. Examples are: Technical performance: bias, repeatability/reproducibility coefficient. Accuracy: Sens, Spec, AUC Biomarkers: change in tumor volume, time to recurrence Patient outcomes: functional status, pain, costs
What do you want to know about θ?	Sometimes we just want to measure θ and put a CI on it; other times we want to test something about θ. Common hypotheses in imaging studies: Superiority hypothesis: $H_o : \theta_{new} = \theta_{old}$; $H_A : \theta_{new} \neq \theta_{old}$ Noninferiority hypothesis: $H_o : \theta_{new} + \delta \leq \theta_{old}$; $H_A : \theta_{new} + \delta > \theta_{old}$
Step 2:	
What is the magnitude of θ?	Sometimes we need an approximate magnitude for θ; other times we can make a conservative guess.
For a superiority hypothesis, what is the clinically relevant difference to detect?	For a superiority hypothesis, the clinically relevant difference is the minimum difference between θ_{new} and θ_{old} that is clinically important to detect
For a noninferiority hypothesis, what is the noninferiority criterion, δ?	For a noninferiority hypothesis, we must define what we mean by "noninferior." If the new modality can by 5% worse than the old modality and still be considered noninferior, then $\delta = 5\%$.
What are the sources of variability in the study and what are their magnitudes?	Depending on the study, there can be many sources of noise, including intra- and interpatient, intra- and interreader, interscanner, intersite
Step 3:	
For constructing a CI, how precise does the CI need to be?	The precision of a CI is usually measured by the half width of the CI
What is the acceptable type I error rate?	When our study data leads us to reject the null hypothesis (H_o) in favor of the alternative hypothesis (H_A), we are making a type I error if H_o was really true. Usually we set the type I error rate at 0.05
What is the acceptable type II error rate*?	When our study data leads us to *not* reject the null hypothesis (H_o), we are making a type II error if H_A was really true. We often set the type II error rate at 0.10 or 0.20

*The complement of the type II error rate is the power. When H_A is true, power equals 1-prob(type II error). If H_A is true, we want to be able to reject H_o in favor $H_{A'}$, so we want high power for our study. Usually we set the power at 0.90 or 0.80.

failure, and dropouts; sample size calculations are complicated even when assumptions are met. Many imaging studies include multiple readers interpreting the same images. The correlation between the readers must be accounted for. Furthermore, we often want to determine both the number of readers and the number of patients needed for the study in order to find a reasonable balance between the two. In Section 7.5.4 we present sample size considerations for an MRMC study.

Investigators often want to get a ballpark estimate of the required sample size before discussing the details with a statistician. Table 7.3 illustrates some simple sample size calculations for different types of research questions that can serve as a first pass. The table also provides a quick reference to the statistical literature for methods that account for the more complicated issues that are common in these studies.

7.5.4 Example sample size considerations for MRMC study

We now illustrate the steps in sample size estimation using Case example 1.1 for illustration. Case example 1.1 is a diagnostic accuracy study, so we use the area under the ROC curve as the primary outcome variable. Our study objective is to estimate readers' area under the ROC curve with the new blood-pool agent (Agent "A") and test whether it is as good as readers' accuracy with the state-of-the-art agent (Agent "B"). Statistically, we state the null and alternative hypotheses as

$$H_o : \theta_A + \delta \leq \theta_B; \ H_A : \theta_A + \delta > \theta_B$$

where θ denotes the readers' mean area under the ROC curve (see Chapter 8 for a full explanation of the types of statistical hypotheses). To test these hypotheses, we must determine an appropriate value for the noninferiority criterion δ. A commonly used criterion for diagnostic accuracy studies is 0.05. Note that larger values for δ (e.g., 0.10) result in a smaller sample size, but the definition of "noninferiority" is more lax (i.e., weak), while smaller values (e.g., 0.01) provide a more stringent criterion and require a larger sample size.

From the literature we would probably have some sense of the value of θ_B, but we should be careful not to overestimate its value because larger values of the area under the ROC curve have smaller variance, leading to smaller sample sizes. In sample size calculations it is important to err on the side of a larger study because of the consequences associated with a low-powered study (see discussion in Section 7.5.1). For illustration, we use 0.80 as the hypothesized value of θ_B.

We also need an estimate of the value of θ_A. There are three options: the new contrast agent will improve readers' accuracy, the new contrast agent will reduce readers' accuracy a little, and the new contrast agent will have no effect on readers' accuracy. We will assume the latter, that is, $\theta_A = 0.8$.

In an MRMC study there are two major sources of variability that we need to consider: the variability among the subjects being imaged and the variability

Table 7.3 Guide to sample size calculations.

Statistical goal	Quick sample size method* and references
Single-arm study:	
Construct 95% CI around Sens (or Spec)	$N_a = \left[1.96 \times \sqrt{p(1-p)}\right]^2 / L^2$, where p is the best guess estimate of the sensitivity, N_a is the number of subjects required with the abnormality, and L is the width of one-half of the CI. This formula assumes one observation/subject. For multiple observations/subject, see Jung et al. [19]
Construct 95% CI around AUC	$N_a = \left[1.96 \times \sqrt{\mathrm{AUC}(1-\mathrm{AUC})}\right]^2 / L^2$, where N_n must be at least as large as N_a. This formula provides a conservative estimate [20]; for other approaches and other summary measures from the ROC curve, see Zhou et al. [2]. For multiple observations/subject, see Obuchowski [21]
Construct 95% CI around a mean (e.g., mean bias)	$N = [1.96 \times \mathrm{SD}]^2 / L^2$, where SD is the standard deviation of the Y_i's
Two-arm study:	
Compare two modalities' Sens (or Spec)	$N_a = \left[\left(z_{1-\alpha} + z_{1-\beta}\right) \times \sqrt{\mathrm{Var}(p_1 - p_2)p_1 - p_2}\right]^2 / (p_1 - p_2)^2$, where p_1 is the best guess estimate of the sensitivity for modality 1 and p_2 is the sensitivity for modality 2, $\mathrm{Var}(p_1 - p_2)$ is the variance of the difference in sensitivities between the two modalities, $z_{1-\alpha}$ is 1.96 for a two-tailed test with 0.05 significance level, and $z_{1-\beta}$ is 0.84 for a study with 80% power. Calculation of the variance depends on the study design. For a paired design, see Lachenbruch [22]. For an unpaired design, $\mathrm{Var}(p_1 - p_2) = p_1 \times (1 - p_1) + p_2 \times (1 - p_2)$. For multiple observations/subject, see Gonen [23]
Compare two modalities' AUC	For a single reader, $N_a = \left[\left(z_{1-\alpha} + z_{1-\beta}\right) \times \sqrt{\mathrm{Var}(\mathrm{AUC}_1 - \mathrm{AUC}_2)}\right]^2 / (\mathrm{AUC}_1 - \mathrm{AUC}_2)^2$, where N_n must be at least as large as N_a. Calculation of the variance depends on the study design. For a paired design, see Zhou et al. [2]. For an unpaired design, a conservative estimate is $\mathrm{Var}(\mathrm{AUC}_1 - \mathrm{AUC}_2) = \mathrm{AUC}_1 \times (1 - \mathrm{AUC}_1) + \mathrm{AUC}_2 \times (1 - \mathrm{AUC}_2)$. For multiple observations/subject, see Obuchowski [21]
Compare two modalities' means (e.g., mean bias)	$N = \left[\left(z_{1-\alpha} + z_{1-\beta}\right) \times \sqrt{\mathrm{Var}(\theta_1 - \theta_2)}\right]^2 / (\theta_1 - \theta_2)^2$, where $\mathrm{Var}(\theta_1 - \theta_2) = \mathrm{Var}(\theta_1) + \mathrm{Var}(\theta_2) - 2 \times r \times \sqrt{\mathrm{Var}(\theta_1) \times \mathrm{Var}(\theta_2)}$, where r is the correlation in the measurements Y_1's and Y_2's. For unpaired designs, $r = 0$
Compare time-to-event in two groups of subjects	See Lachin and Foulkes [24] and Schoenfeld [25]
MRMC study:	
Compare two modalities' AUC from MRMC† study	See Zhou et al. [2] for formula and definitions. See Section 7.5.4 for an example. See Obuchowski [26] for sample size tables for studies with one observation/subject and Obuchowski and Hillis [27] for tables with multiple observations/subject. For determining sample size from pilot data, see Hillis et al. [28]. For MRMC noninferiority studies, see Chen et al. [29]

*Methods presented are for CI construction and superiority hypotheses. See Blackwelder [30] for noninferiority designs.
†MRMC, multireader multicase.

among the readers interpreting the images. We denote these as σ_c^2 (variability due to cases, or subjects) and σ_r^2 (variability due to readers). A commonly used estimate of σ_c^2 [31] is

$$\hat{\sigma}_c^2 = \left(0.0099 \times e^{-A \times A/2}\right) \times \frac{\left[\left(5A^2 + 8\right) + \left(A^2 + 8\right)/k\right]}{N_a}$$

where A is a parameter from the ROC curve, k is the ratio of normal to abnormal subjects in the study sample (i.e., $k = N_n/N_a$), and N_a is the number of subjects with an abnormality in the study sample. The total sample size for the study is $N_a(1+k)$. For AUC values of 0.7, 0.8, and 0.9, a reasonable estimate of A for sample size estimation is 0.74, 1.19, and 1.82, respectively [2]. If we were planning a prospective study, the prevalence of disease would likely be low, say, 10% for illustration; then $k = 9/1 = 9$. For a retrospective study, we might choose to select equal numbers of subjects with and without the abnormality; thus $k = 1$. Then, for our example,

$$\hat{\sigma}_c^2 = \left(0.0099 \times e^{-1.19 \times 1.19/2}\right) \times \frac{\left[\left(5\{1.19\}^2 + 8\right) + \left(\{1.19\}^2 + 8\right)/k\right]}{N_a}$$

which equals $0.11946/N_a$ for $k = 1$ and $0.07865/N_a$ for $k = 9$.

Note that we are assuming one observation per subject. If there are multiple observations from the same subject (e.g., multiple liver lesions), then we must adjust N_a to reflect this. A simple approach is to guestimate the average number of observations per subject (call it s) and guestimate the correlation between observations from the same subject (call it r). For example, in Case example 1.1 we might assume an average of two liver metastases per subject with metastases. Often the correlation between observations from the same subject is moderate [27], so we might set $r = 0.5$. Then the **effective sample size** is $[N_a \times s]/[(1+(s-1) \times r)]$. In Case example 1.1, the effective sample size is $[N_a \times 2]/1.5$. Note that if there was no correlation ($r = 0$) between lesions from the same subject, the effective sample size would be $N_a \times 2$. If the lesions from the same subject were perfectly correlated ($r = 1$), then the effective sample size would be N_a. This makes intuitive sense because the more correlated the observations from the same subject are, the less information they provide for our study.

To estimate the variability between readers, we might postulate the range of readers' ROC areas. For Agent B, perhaps the literature suggests that readers' AUCs will be as low as 0.7 and as high as 0.9. Then with some underlying assumptions about the distribution [2], we estimate $\hat{\sigma}_r^2 = [(\text{range})/4]^2$. For our example, $\hat{\sigma}_r^2 = [(0.9-0.7)/4]^2 = 0.0025$.

The next step in our sample size calculation requires consideration of the study design. Zhou et al. [2] and Obuchowski [32] describe various options for MRMC study designs. For illustration, we will consider the most commonly used MRMC design, whereby the same subjects are imaged with all modalities being studied (i.e., the subjects are imaged with the standard agent on one day and with the new agent on a different day) and all of the readers interpret the study images from both agents. This design is referred to as a paired reader, paired subject design. With this design, we must consider the magnitude of the correlations produced from the pairings. The correlation r_1 describes the correlation due to the paired subject design. For an unpaired subject design, r_1 will equal zero, but for a paired design investigators often set $r_1 = 0.5$ for sample size estimation [2]. There are two other correlations, r_2 and r_3, that exist in an MRMC-paired subject design. These two correlations are often similar in magnitude; thus for sample size purposes investigators set them equal to each other [33].

The correlation r_b describes the correlation due to the paired reader design. For an unpaired reader design, r_b will equal zero, but for a paired reader design, $r_b > 0$. Its value can vary considerably depending on the experience of the readers with each of the modalities being studied. If the most accurate readers on one modality will likely be the most accurate on other modalities, then r_b is large. If readers have different experiences with interpreting images from the different modalities, then r_b may be smaller. For illustration, we assume that readers who are the most accurate with the old contrast agent will also be most accurate with the new agent; thus we set $r_b = 0.75$.

A formula for determining power for an MRMC study is

$$\lambda = \frac{R\left(\left(\theta_A - \theta_B\right) + \delta\right)^2}{2\left\{\sigma_r^2\left(1 - r_b\right) + \sigma_c^2\left[\left(1 - r_1\right)\right]\right\}}$$

where R is the number of readers in the study. λ is the called the noncentrality parameter. Various statistical and mathematical packages will calculate the study's power based on the value of λ, using the noncentral F-distribution with degrees of freedom equal to $(I\text{-}1)$ and $(R\text{-}1)$ for comparing I modalities in a study with R readers (see R language, SAS, MATLAB, Mathematica, NumPy, and Boost C++ libraries).

Figure 7.5 illustrates the number of readers (x-axis) versus the number of subjects (y-axis) needed for Case example 1.1 with 80% power and 5% type I error rate. The two curves represent two designs: blue is a retrospective study with $k = 0.5$ and red is a prospective study with $k = 9$. Designs with more subjects require fewer readers, although the relationship is not linear. For example, a prospective study could be carried out with 620 total subjects (i.e., 62 with the abnormality and 558 without) and 10 readers, or with 280 subjects and 15 readers. A retrospective study would require 190 subjects (95 with the abnormality and 95 without) and 10 readers or 84 subjects and 15 readers. The retrospective design requires smaller sample sizes because k is set at an optimal level of one. A design with fewer subjects is desirable when it is expensive or difficult to recruit subjects. In contrast, a design with more subjects (fewer readers) should be chosen if there are subject characteristics that affect test accuracy (i.e., lesion size and location) so that precise estimates of accuracy can be calculated for these important subpopulations.

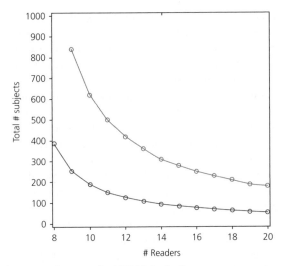

Figure 7.5 Sample size requirements for MRMC Study. Top curve represents prospective design; bottom curve depicts retrospective design.

References

1 Roland, M. and D.J. Torgerson, Understanding controlled trials: what are pragmatic trials? *BMJ*, 1998. **316**(7127): p. 285.

2 Zhou, X., N.A. Obuchowski, and D.K. McClish, *Statistical Methods in Diagnostic Medicine, 2nd ed.* 2011, John Wiley & Sons, Inc.: Hoboken, NJ.

3 Thornbury, J.R., et al., Disk-caused nerve compression in patients with acute low-back pain: diagnosis with MR, CT myelography, and plain CT. *Radiology*, 1993. **186**(3): p. 731–738.

4 de Graaff, J.C., et al., The diagnostic randomized clinical trial is the best solution for management issues in critical limb ischemia. *J Clin Epidemiol*, 2004. **57**(11): p. 1111–1118.

5 Lijmer, J.G. and P.M.M. Bossuyt, Various randomized designs can be used to evaluate medical tests. *J Clin Epidemiol*, 2009. **62**(4): p. 364–373.

6 Obuchowski, N.A. and X.-H. Zhou, Prospective studies of diagnostic test accuracy when disease prevalence is low. *Biostatistics*, 2002. **3**(4): p. 477–492.

7 Freedman, B., Equipoise and the ethics of clinical research. *N Engl J Med*, 1987. **317**(3): p. 141–145.

8 Bossuyt, P.M., J.G. Lijmer, and B.W. Mol, Randomised comparisons of medical tests: sometimes invalid, not always efficient. *Lancet*, 2000. **356**(9244): p. 1844–1847.

9 Lu, B. and C. Gatsonis, Efficiency of study designs in diagnostic randomized clinical trials. *Stat Med*, 2013. **32**(9): p. 1451–1466.

10 Pocock, S.J., Group sequential methods in the design and analysis of clinical trials. *Biometrika*, 1977. **64**(2): p. 191–199.

11 O'Brien, P.C. and T.R. Fleming, A multiple testing procedure for clinical trials. *Biometrics*, 1979. **35**(3): p. 549–556.

12 Barker, A.D., et al., I-SPY 2: an adaptive breast cancer trial design in the setting of neoadjuvant chemotherapy. *Clin Pharmacol Ther*, 2009. **86**(1): p. 97–100.

13 Chin, R., *Adaptive and Flexible Clinical Trials.* 2012, Chapman & Hall/CRC: Boca Raton, FL.

14 Chow, S. and M. Chang, *Adaptive Design Methods in Clinical Trials (2 ed.)*, 2012, Chapman & Hall/CRC: Boca Raton, FL.

15 Jennison, C. and B. Turnbull, *Group Sequential Methods with Applications to Clinical Trials*. 1999, Chapman & Hall/CRC: Boca Raton, FL.

16 Whitehead, J., Stopping clinical trials by design. *Nat Rev Drug Discov*, 2004. **3**(11): p. 973–977.

17 Kukull, W.A. and M. Ganguli, Generalizability: the trees, the forest, and the low-hanging fruit. *Neurology*, 2012. **78**(23): p. 1886–1891.

18 Jarvik, J.G., et al., Rapid magnetic resonance imaging vs radiographs for patients with low back pain: a randomized controlled trial. *JAMA*, 2003. **289**(21): p. 2810–2818.

19 Jung, S.H., S.H. Kang, and C. Ahn, Sample size calculations for clustered binary data. *Stat Med*, 2001. **20**(13): p. 1971–1982.

20 Blume, J.D., Bounding sample size projections for the area under a ROC curve. *J Stat Plann Inference*, 2009. **139**(1): p. 711–721.

21 Obuchowski, N.A., Nonparametric analysis of clustered ROC curve data. *Biometrics*, 1997. **53**(2): p. 567–578.

22 Lachenbruch, P.A., On the sample size for studies based upon McNemar's test. *Stat Med*, 1992. **11**(11): p. 1521–1525.

23 Gonen, M., Sample size and power for McNemar's test with clustered data. *Stat Med*, 2004. **23**(14): p. 2283–2294.

24 Lachin, J.M. and M.A. Foulkes, Evaluation of sample size and power for analyses of survival with allowance for nonuniform patient entry, losses to follow-up, noncompliance, and stratification. *Biometrics*, 1986. **42**(3): p. 507–519.

25 Schoenfeld, D.A., Sample-size formula for the proportional-hazards regression model. *Biometrics*, 1983. **39**(2): p. 499–503.

26 Obuchowski, N.A., Sample size tables for receiver operating characteristic studies. *AJR Am J Roentgenol*, 2000. **175**(3): p. 603–608.

27 Obuchowski, N.A. and S.L. Hillis, Sample size tables for computer-aided detection studies. *AJR Am J Roentgenol*, 2011. **197**(5): p. 821–828.

28 Hillis, S.L., N.A. Obuchowski, and K.S. Berbaum, Power estimation for multireader ROC methods an updated and unified approach. *Acad Radiol*, 2011. **18**(2): p. 129–142.

29 Chen, W., N.A. Petrick, and B. Sahiner, Hypothesis testing in noninferiority and equivalence MRMC ROC studies. *Acad Radiol*, 2012. **19**(9): p. 1158–1165.

30 Blackwelder, W.C., "Proving the null hypothesis" in clinical trials. *Control Clin Trials*, 1982. **3**(4): p. 345–353.

31 Obuchowski, N.A. and D.K. McClish, Sample size determination for diagnostic accuracy studies involving binormal ROC curve indices. *Stat Med*, 1997. **16**(13): p. 1529–1542.

32 Obuchowski, N.A., Reducing the number of reader interpretations in MRMC studies. *Acad Radiol*, 2009. **16**(2): p. 209–217.

33 Rockette, H.E., et al., Empiric assessment of parameters that affect the design of multireader receiver operating characteristic studies. *Acad Radiol*, 1999. **6**(12): p. 723–729.

CHAPTER 8

Introduction to biostatistical methods

Diana L. Miglioretti[1], Todd A. Alonzo[2] and Nancy A. Obuchowski[3]

[1] *University of California Davis School of Medicine, Davis, CA, USA*
[2] *University of Southern California, Los Angeles, CA, USA*
[3] *Quantitative Health Sciences, Cleveland Clinic Foundation, Cleveland, OH, USA*

KEY POINTS

- The first step in a statistical analysis is to summarize data using descriptive and exploratory analyses.

- A summary statistic, such as a mean, should always be reported with a measure of precision, such as a confidence interval.

- Statistical hypothesis testing provides a formal framework for determining whether a pattern observed in the sample data is unlikely to have occurred by chance alone.

- Study designs should consider two types of possible errors in hypothesis testing, type I and type II errors.

8.1 Role of biostatistics in clinical imaging research

Why is biostatistics important for radiologists? Biostatistics provides a way to formally evaluate evidence, rather than relying on anecdotal experiences. Biostatistics helps us find patterns in the uncertainty inherent to radiology practice due to variability in the patients seen and the interpretations made. It provides the tools we need to determine whether these patterns are likely reflective of true patterns in the underlying population or explained by chance. Radiologists rely on qualitative and quantitative data to make diagnoses. It is important to understand the accuracy of these diagnoses to optimize care. Last, an understanding of biostatistics provides the knowledge needed to critically evaluate the literature.

Clinical imaging research involves the following steps:
1 Formalizing the research question including developing testable hypotheses
2 Collecting and evaluating relevant data from the population of interest

---

Handbook for Clinical Trials of Imaging and Image-Guided Interventions, First Edition.
Edited by Nancy A. Obuchowski and G. Scott Gazelle.
© 2016 John Wiley & Sons, Inc. Published 2016 by John Wiley & Sons, Inc.

3 Exploring systematic patterns versus random variation in these data
4 Weighing the strength of patterns relative to variation
5 Accepting or rejecting of a priori hypotheses concerning relationships
6 Interpreting and communicating results

Biostatistics has an important role in each of these steps. It helps us determine how we can best collect data, how we should analyze those data, and what inferences we can make from those data. Biostatistics allows researchers to use a **statistic**, which is a function of data collected on the sample, to estimate a population parameter.

In this chapter, we provide an introduction to biostatistics to help you:

- Summarize data using descriptive and exploratory analyses
- Understand measures of central tendency and variation
- Translate clinical research questions to statistical (testable) hypotheses
- Understand two types of errors in hypothesis testing (type I and type II)
- Interpret p-values

8.2 Descriptive and exploratory data analysis

Once a study is conducted and data are collected, the first step of an analysis is to look at the data, one variable at a time [1]. This process generally involves:

1 Initial summarization of data, including checking for unusual or erroneous values and identifying missing items
2 Descriptive and exploratory analysis of data
3 Preliminary interpretation of data

The techniques used in (1–3) are collectively called **exploratory data analysis** (EDA).

A dataset for a research study is typically organized as one row per observation and one column per variable. An **observation** is a unique item of information on a unit of interest, such as a patient or physician. A **variable** is a quantity measured on each observation that may vary from observation to observation. A variable may be either:

- **Qualitative**, if the values are categorical or
- **Quantitative**, if the values are intrinsically numeric

A qualitative variable with only two possible categories, such as the presence or absence of a finding or a patient's disease status, is called **binary**. It is difficult to analyze free text fields, so it is recommended to use coded, numeric values rather than text fields. For example, a binary variable may be given the value of 1 (i.e., positive or "success") if the event or category of primary interest is observed or given the value of 0 (i.e., negative or "failure") if the other possible category is observed. A qualitative variable with more than two categories may be either **nominal**, if there is no intrinsic ordering (e.g., race or country of birth, modality type), or **ordinal**, if the categories can be ranked, such as a mild, moderate, or severe finding on an image. Again, when creating a study dataset, observed values

Table 8.1 Sample observations from dataset.

Subject	Reference standard	Imaging method	Confidence score	Stone size (mm)
1	0	0	0	0
1	0	1	0	0
2	1	0	4	3
2	1	1	4	3
3	0	0	0	0
3	0	1	3	0
4	1	0	4	2
4	1	1	4	2
...	...	...	...	...
50	1	0	4	5
50	1	1	4	5

for nominal and ordinal variables should be coded as numbers instead of free text for analysis. A codebook or **data dictionary** should be created to document the value each code represents.

A quantitative variable is considered **discrete** if it has a finite number of possible values, such as the number of nodules on a lung CT. **Continuous** quantitative variables can take an infinite number of possible values, such as the size of a finding on an image or a patient's survival time following treatment.

Consider a study comparing two computed tomographic (CT) imaging methods for detecting renal stones: the standard 100% exposure images reconstructed with filtered back projection (FBP) and a new 50% exposure image reconstructed with sinogram-affirmed iterative reconstruction called SAFIRE. The scientific question is whether radiologists are able to detect renal stones using the lower-dose image as well as when using the traditional image taken with full radiation exposure. Table 8.1 shows a sample of five observations from the study dataset with 100 observations from 50 subjects (each subject contributes two records) [2]. The reference standard is binary, coded as either 0 (no renal stones present) or 1 (renal stones present). The imaging method is also binary, coded here as 0 for FBP CT or 1 for SAFIRE, the new lower-dose CT with reconstructed images. The confidence score is an ordinal categorical variable taking the following possible values: 0=definitely no renal stone, 1=probably no renal stone, 2=possibly a renal stone, 3=probably a renal stone, and 4=definitely a renal stone. We consider a stone to be *detected* if it was given a score of 3 or more. The stone size is a continuous variable that could potentially take an infinite number of possible values but is shown here to the nearest millimeter.

8.2.1 Summary statistics
An important part of starting the data analysis process is familiarizing yourself with the data and identifying possible errors and anomalies. The goal is data reduction while preserving and extracting key information about the process

Table 8.2 Distribution of confidence score by imaging modality and reference standard.

Confidence Score	Patients with a stone				Patients without a stone			
	FBP		SAFIRE		FBP		SAFIRE	
	N	(%)	N	(%)	N	(%)	N	(%)
0	1	5	1	5	27	93	21	72
1	0	0	1	5	1	3	2	7
2	0	0	0	0	0	0	1	3
3	3	14	3	14	1	3	5	17
4	17	81	16	76	0	0	0	0

under investigation. A simple and effective way to summarize qualitative (i.e., categorical) variables is to tabulate the **frequency distribution**, which shows the number and percentage of observations in each category.

Frequency distributions can also be created for qualitative variables by grouping the data into a finite number of categories. The association between multiple categorical variables can be explored using cross-tabulations, showing row and/or column percentages. For example, Table 8.2 shows the distribution of the confidence scores by imaging modality and the reference standard for the renal stone dataset. Of the 21 subjects with renal stones, 20 (95%) were detected using FBP and 19 (90%) were detected using SAFIRE. Of the 29 patients without renal stones, 1 (3%) was falsely considered to have stones on FBP and 5 (17%) on SAFIRE.

For quantitative variables, it is important to explore the sample distribution before computing summary statistics. We discuss graphical displays in Section 8.2.2. Important summary statistics include measures of central tendency and measures of dispersion. These are discussed in the next couple of subsections.

8.2.1.1 Measures of central tendency

The center of a distribution is typically summarized by the mean, median, and/or mode. The arithmetic **mean**, $\bar{Y}$, is the most commonly used and is the sum of all the observations divided by the sample size (N):

$$\bar{Y} = \frac{\sum_i^N Y_i}{N}.$$

In other words, the mean is the simple average of the observations.

Imaging studies commonly collect binary data, for example, the result of an imaging test may be assessed as *positive* or *negative*. The mean of a binary variable is a **proportion** [3]. For example, the sensitivity and specificity of a test are proportions.

The mean is intuitive and frequently used; however, outliers (i.e., observations that are much larger or smaller than most values) and skewness (i.e., asymmetry in the distribution) can influence it. For skewed distributions, the **median**, or middle value, may better represent the central tendency. If there are an odd number of observations, the median is simply the middle value when the data are ordered from low to high. If there is an even number of observations, then it is the average of two middle values. The **mode** is the most common value observed. Sometimes a population may have more than one mode.

8.2.1.2 Measures of dispersion

Variability is also important [4]! It is important to understand how dispersed observations in a population are from the center of the distribution. For example, for Case example 1.2, it is important to understand how much ^{18}F-FDG uptake varies within responders and within nonresponders. In addition, each study sample will be different, and it is important to understand how samples vary from each other when making inferences. Variation is small if observations are bunched near the mean and is large if observations are widely scattered. A simple measure of dispersion is the **range**, which is the largest value minus the smallest value. The **interquartile range** (IQR) is the middle 50% of the data, that is, the 75th percentile minus the 25th percentile. The range and IQR only depend on two numbers. The **variance** measures the average of the (squared) distances of the observations from the mean:

$$\mathrm{Var}(Y) = \frac{\sum_{i=1}^{N}(Y_i - \bar{Y})^2}{N-1}.$$

The differences between the observations and the mean are squared before summing so the negative deviations do not cancel out the positive deviations. The justification for dividing by $N-1$ instead of N is beyond the scope of this introductory book. In brief, $N-1$ is the **degrees of freedom**, which is a measure of how much information is in the sample. Simply put, we lose one degree of freedom for estimating the mean; thus, there are $N-1$ pieces of information remaining for estimating the variance.

The variance is a function of the square of the deviations from the mean; thus the units are in the square of the units of the observations. The **standard deviation** (SD) puts the measure in the same units as the observations by taking the square root of the variance:

$$\mathrm{SD}(Y) = \sqrt{\mathrm{Var}(Y)} = \sqrt{\frac{\sum_{i=1}^{N}(Y_i - \bar{Y})^2}{N-1}}.$$

The **standard error** (SE) **of the mean** measures the precision of the estimated mean. It is the SD divided by the square root of the sample size:

$$\mathrm{SE}(\bar{Y}) = \frac{\mathrm{SD}(Y)}{\sqrt{N}}.$$

The variance of a proportion p is simply $p(1-p)$; thus, the **SE of a proportion** estimated from N observations is

$$SE(p) = \sqrt{\frac{p(1-p)}{N}}.$$

Unlike the SD, the SE gets smaller as the sample size gets larger. Thus, the SE is typically much smaller than the SD. It is important to understand the difference between the SD and the SE. The SD measures variability in the data, that is, how much the individual observations deviate from the population mean. The SE measures the precision of the sample mean in estimating the true population mean, that is, how much the mean estimated from a single sample might deviate from the true population mean.

8.2.1.3 Confidence intervals

Providing a sample estimate, for example, a mean or proportion, alone without information on variability is not very useful to a researcher. Thus, it is important to always include a measure of precision with a summary statistic. Typically, a **confidence interval** should be provided, because it shows a range of values that are likely to encompass the actual ("true") population value. Wider confidence intervals indicate lesser precision of the estimate; narrower confidence intervals indicate greater precision. Under frequentist statistics (vs. Bayesian statistics), the exact interpretation of a confidence interval is

> If repeated samples of size N are obtained from the population and a 95% confidence interval constructed for each sample, then 95% of the constructed confidence intervals are expected to include the true population value and 5% are not.

Unfortunately, we have no way of knowing whether the confidence interval estimated from our single study sample includes the true value or not! Figure 8.1 demonstrates this using a small simulation study. The blue intervals contain the true mean, which is 0. The red intervals do not. On average, about 5% of the intervals will be red—they will not contain the true mean. Unfortunately, we typically only get to see one of these confidence intervals from our study, and we have no way of knowing if our confidence interval is one of the blue or red ones, that is, if it contains the true mean or not.

It is important to understand that the percentage of intervals that don't contain the true mean is independent of the sample size! As the sample size grows, the confidence interval gets smaller, meaning the estimated mean is more precise. However, on average, 5% of those confidence intervals will still not include the true mean. In Figure 8.1, we see that approximately 5% of the intervals do not contain the true mean for either the small samples of size 12 or the large samples of size 100.

When calculating a confidence interval, we often rely on the **central limit theorem**, which says that for a sufficiently large sample of independent observations, the sample mean will be approximately normally distributed, regardless of

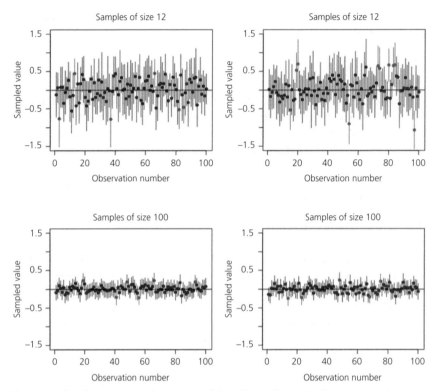

Figure 8.1 Plots demonstrating that 95% confidence intervals contain the true mean for approximately 95% of study samples, regardless of the sample size. For each plot, we simulated 100 samples of either 12 or 100 observations from a normal distribution with a mean of 0 and a standard deviation of 1. The black intervals contain the true mean, which is 0. The gray intervals do not.

the underlying distribution. When the underlying distribution is not strongly skewed, a sample of at least 30 observations is typically large enough for the sample mean to be approximately normal. For very skewed distributions, the central limit theorem still holds, but larger sample sizes are required for the sampling distribution of the mean to be approximately normal.

Using the central limit theorem, the 95% confidence interval for the mean, $\bar{Y}$, can be calculated as

$$\bar{Y} \pm 1.96 \frac{\text{SD}}{\sqrt{N}}.$$

The value 1.96 in this equation comes from a normal distribution—for normally distributed data, 95% of the values fall within ±1.96 SD of the mean. A 90% confidence interval can be constructed by replacing 1.96 with 1.645 in the above formula.

For a proportion p, we can also rely on the central limit theorem if p is estimated from a large enough sample. The sample size needed for the normality assumption to be reasonable for calculating a confidence interval for a proportion depends on how rare the event is, that is, the value of p. Typically, the normality assumption will be reasonable if we expect at least 10 *successes* (i.e., positives) and 10 *failures* (i.e., negatives) in our sample, that is, $Np \geq 10$ and $N(1-p) \geq 10$. In this case, the 95% confidence interval can be calculated as

$$p \pm 1.96 \sqrt{\frac{p(1-p)}{N}}.$$

If this **success–failure condition** is not met, other methods for calculating confidence intervals for proportions may be more appropriate [5].

8.2.2 Graphs

Graphical displays are very effective for descriptive analysis of both categorical and numeric data [1]. Useful graphs communicate complex ideas clearly, precisely, and efficiently. Good graphs show the most amount of information with the least amount of ink in the smallest space [6]. In general, pie charts are not very useful because they are hard to read, use a lot of ink to show a small amount of information, and are difficult to compare across multiple groups.

The most common graph for exploring and summarizing categorical data is the **bar chart**. A bar chart shows the number or percentage of observations in each category. The horizontal axis shows the different categories, and the height of each bar represents the frequency of observations in that category. The bars should be separated from each other, so it is clear the categories are separate and not continuous. For example, Figure 8.2 shows the distributions of confidence scores from FBP versus SAFIRE for cases with stones.

For quantitative data, several types of plots are useful for EDA:

1 **Histograms** are helpful for visualizing the shape of the distribution. The horizontal axis corresponds to the range of the quantitative variables, divided into

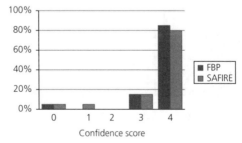

Figure 8.2 Bar chart showing the distribution of confidence scores from FBP versus SAFIRE for cases with stones.

bins or categories. The vertical axis shows the frequency (count in each category), relative frequency (proportion in each category), or percentage in the bins. Bars of the correct height, with adjacent bars touching to indicate the continuity, show the distribution. Histograms may be used to examine the center, spread, and shape of the distribution. Bin sizes should be selected so that the distribution is smooth but important features of the distribution are maintained. Figure 8.3 shows a histogram of the distribution of the radiation dose from over 10,000 abdominal CT, nicely illustrating that the distribution is positively (right) skewed.

2 **Boxplots** are also useful for summarizing quantitative data and may be better than histograms for visually comparing two or more distributions. The box shows the middle 50% of the data, which is the IQR (the lower to the upper quartile). The horizontal line within the box corresponds to the median. The whiskers go out 1.5 box widths or to last point inside that range. Values past that "fence" are potential outliers. Figure 8.4 illustrates boxplots of the distribution of the radiation doses from abdominal CT examinations performed before and after an intervention aimed at optimizing doses. It shows the median did not change, but the variability decreased, especially for the higher values, after the intervention.

3 **Stem-and-leaf plots** can be helpful for exploring small datasets because actual values of observations are shown. The stem-and-leaf display is like a sideways histogram—only the bars are populated with the actual digits. The "stem" is the leading digit or digits, shown on the left. On each stem, the final digit for each observation is shown as a "leaf." Figure 8.5 illustrates a histogram of the distribution of the radiation dose from 100 randomly selected abdominal CT exams.

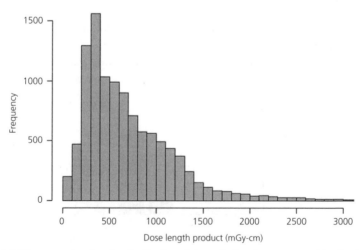

Figure 8.3 Histogram showing the distribution of the radiation dose, measured by the dose length product, from over 10,000 abdominal CT exams.

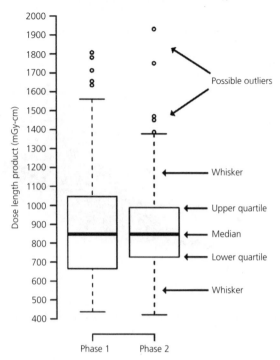

Figure 8.4 Boxplots showing the distribution of the radiation dose, measured by the dose length product, from abdominal CT exams performed before (phase 1) and after (phase 2) an intervention aimed at optimizing doses.

```
The decimal point is 2 digit(s) to the right of the |

 1 | 89
 2 | 00024467789
 3 | 2236667788889
 4 | 1112223447
 5 | 00124566667779
 6 | 2568
 7 | 022366
 8 | 3578
 9 | 00235
10 | 00333789
11 | 01558
12 | 24789
13 | 02257
14 | 7
15 | 4
16 |
17 |
18 |
19 | 33
20 |
21 | 45
22 | 9
23 |
24 | 1
```

Figure 8.5 Stem-and-leaf plot showing the distribution of the radiation dose, measured by the dose length product, for 100 randomly selected abdominal CT exams.

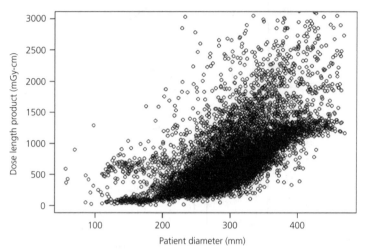

Figure 8.6 Illustrates a scatterplot of radiation dose, measured by the dose length product, by the diameter of the patient's abdomen from over 10,000 abdominal CT exams.

There are two decimal places to the right of the dash, which means the data are rounded to the nearest 10. The smallest two values have a "1" for the leading digit (on the stem) and an "8" and "9" to the right, on the "leaf"—meaning the rounded values are 180 and 190. The maximum value is 2410.

4 **Scatterplots** are very useful for showing the association between two continuous variables. Each observation is plotted as a single dot or other symbols. The value of one variable determines the position on the horizontal axis, and the value of the other variable determines the position of the vertical axis. Figure 8.6 illustrates a scatterplot of radiation dose by the diameter of the patient's abdomen from over 10,000 abdominal CT exams. Dose tends to increase with body size, but doses are still quite variable even for a given body size.

8.3 Confirmatory data analysis (i.e., hypothesis testing)

Recall that a parameter is an unknown characteristic of a population. We cannot know the value of a population parameter; however, we can make inferences about the parameter from our study sample, a subset of the population of interest. Statistical hypothesis testing provides a formal framework for making statistical inference about a population from the data collected on a sample of that population. It is a method for determining whether a pattern observed in the sample data is unlikely to have occurred by chance alone, according to a predetermined level of significance that corresponds to the probability of a chance finding. Statistical hypothesis testing is sometimes called **confirmatory data analysis**, in contrast to **EDA** discussed in Section 8.2.

The steps in statistical hypothesis testing are as follows:

1 Formulate the null (H_0) and alternative (H_A) statistical hypotheses from the clinical question.
2 Specify the significance level, typically 0.05.
3 Collect study data and compute the test statistic.
4 Calculate the resulting **p-value**, which is the probability of observing what you observed or something more extreme if the null hypothesis is true.
5 Decide to either reject or not reject the null hypothesis, H_0:
   - Reject H_0 if the p-value is less than the prespecified level of significance (α; typically 0.05).
   - Do not reject H_0 if the p-value is greater than the significance level. If the p-value is not less than the prespecified significance level, then the evidence is insufficient to reject the null hypothesis. This does not mean we accept the null hypothesis.
6 Interpret result according to the clinical question corresponding to the null hypothesis (H_0), the alternative hypothesis (H_A), and the study population.

We discuss each of these steps in more detail in the following text.

8.3.1 Formulating the null and alternative hypotheses

This first step in statistical hypothesis testing is to formulate the null (H_0) and alternative (H_A) statistical hypotheses from the clinical question. In Chapter 7 we discussed turning a clinical question of interest into testable statistical hypotheses. The null hypothesis is typically worded such that there is no effect or no difference between the population parameters of interest. For example, if testing the accuracy of a new modality, the null hypothesis might state that the accuracy is no better than chance or that it is no better than some minimal level of accuracy necessary to move on to invest in larger studies. Consider the Case example 1.1 introduced in Chapter 1 on evaluating the diagnostic accuracy of a new liver blood-pool agent for detecting colorectal metastases at CT. The null hypothesis might be that Agent A and Agent B are equally accurate for identifying liver metastases from colorectal cancer. A researcher's goal is typically to provide enough evidence to reject the null hypothesis, for example, to show that a new modality is more accurate than the current modality. The alternative hypothesis is typically worded such that there is an effect or a difference in the population parameters in either direction, for example, that one modality is more accurate than another at diagnosing a disease. However, there are other possible designs, discussed in Chapter 7 and Section 8.3.3.

8.3.2 Significance level, test statistics, and *p*-values

P-values are widely reported in the literature but are often poorly understood. The p-value is an estimate of a probability, but may not be the probability you think it is [7]! Say, you develop a new imaging modality and conduct a study because you want to know if your new modality is better than the standard modality. You find that the sensitivity for your new modality is 0.95, which appears to be better than the old modality's sensitivity of 0.90. For the **p-value**, we calculate the probability that we would observe a result at least as extreme as the result we observed if there was truly no difference between the tests (i.e., under the null hypothesis). This may seem backward! Let's try to understand why we calculate the p-value under the assumption of "no difference" if we are looking for a difference in outcome.

Imagine there is a skeptical scientist who does not believe the new modality is better than the standard modality. You and the skeptical scientist review the strength of the evidence pointing toward the alternative hypothesis, using probability models. Then you draw conclusions from this evidence. Sometimes these conclusions might be wrong!

There are two types of errors that could be made (see Table 8.3). For a **type I error**, the skeptic is right, and there truly is no difference between the modalities. The difference you found occurred by chance alone. However, you rejected the null hypothesis of no difference and publish a high-profile article stating your new modality is more sensitive than the conventional modality. Facilities purchase this new modality and change clinical practice because of your research. This would typically be a bad outcome and hard to undo. On the other hand, you could make a **type II error**. In this case, the skeptic is wrong, and your new modality is more sensitive, but you found no difference. You publish your result and miss the chance to improve clinical practice. The severity of this outcome depends on how big of an improvement you missed.

Studies should be designed to control the probability of making these errors by chance. We control the probability of type I error by setting a limit on how high a chance of this we are willing to take. We call this limit the **significance level** and denote it as α (alpha). Alpha (α) is the maximum allowable probability of a type I error. It is prespecified by the investigator and is often, but not always, set to 0.05. We control the probability of a type I error by rejecting the null hypothesis only when the probability that a sample would give this extreme a result or more extreme if the null hypothesis is true and is less than alpha.

The probability of a type II error is usually written as β (beta). To control the type II error, we usually think in terms of $1-\beta$, also called the **power**. The power

Table 8.3 Defining type I and II errors.

		Underlying truth	
		H₀ true	*H₀* false
Decision	Do not reject H_0	Correct decision	Type II error (β)
	Reject H_0	Type I error (α)	Correct decision

is the probability that we reject the null hypothesis when the alternative hypothesis is true. The power depends on the size of the difference, or effect. Note the probability of a type II error decreases, and the power correspondingly increases, with increasing sample size; however, the Type I error is 0.05 regardless of sample size. The choice of statistical procedure can also affect power. You control the type II error, β, by prespecifying your desired power for a given, clinically meaningful, effect and planning the study to attain this (see Chapter 7 for discussion of sample size).

The types of errors made in hypothesis testing are similar to possible errors in diagnostic testing (see Table 8.4). As in diagnostic testing, there is a trade-off between the type I and type II errors. If you reduce α in a fixed-design study, then you usually end up increasing β. Similarly, to decrease the false-negative rate of a diagnostic test, you typically have to increase the false-positive rate.

To calculate a p-value, we need the following:

1 A test statistic, calculated from the data, that reflects the state of nature to discern between the alternative hypothesis (H_A) and the null hypothesis (H_0). The test statistic is typically computed from the sample mean $\bar{Y}$, the sample size N, and the variability of the sample statistic (such as the SE of the mean, $SE(\bar{Y})$).
2 A probability model for the test statistic if the null hypothesis was true.
3 A way to calculate the probability of a test statistic value at least as extreme as what we observe, if the null hypothesis (H_0) is true. This probability is called the p-value.

The appropriate test statistic and probability model will depend on the hypotheses being tested, the outcome being studied, and the analytic method being used [8–10]. Due to the central limit theorem, many test statistics used in imaging studies, for example, tests comparing sensitivities, specificities, and ROC area under the curve, follow a normal distribution. To test the null hypothesis that two means $\bar{Y}_1$ and $\bar{Y}_2$ (or proportions) from two independent groups of subjects (Group 1 and Group 2) are equal, one can calculate the following z statistic:

$$z = \frac{\bar{Y}_1 - \bar{Y}_2}{\sqrt{\dfrac{\text{Var}(\bar{Y}_1)}{N_1} + \dfrac{\text{Var}(\bar{Y}_2)}{N_2}}}$$

Table 8.4 Comparing false negative and positive rates to type I and II errors.

		True disease status	
		Disease	**No disease**
Test result	Positive	Correct decision	False positive
	Negative	False negative	Correct decision

where Var($\overline{Y}_1$) is the variance for the N_1 participants in Group 1 and Var($\overline{Y}_2$) is the variance for the N_2 participants in Group 2. The value of z can be compared with the standard normal distribution to obtain a p-value.

8.3.3 Types of hypothesis tests

There are four types of hypothesis tests typically used in imaging research:

1 *Test for difference*—To demonstrate a difference between two imaging modalities by rejecting the null hypothesis of no difference when the alternative hypothesis states the new modality is either superior or inferior to the traditional modality.

2 *Superiority test*—To demonstrate superiority of one imaging modality versus another by rejecting the null hypothesis of no difference when the alternative hypothesis states the new modality is superior.

3 *Equivalence test*—To show that two imaging modalities differ by no more than a prespecified amount (the equivalence margin).

4 *Noninferiority test*—To show that a new imaging modality is not worse than a standard modality by more than the noninferiority margin.

8.3.3.1 Test for difference

Often, we are interested in testing whether two population parameters (e.g., the accuracy of two imaging modalities) are different. For example, suppose we want to compare the sensitivity of CT with Agent A versus Agent B for identifying liver metastases from colorectal cancer, as in Case example 1.1. In this situation, we frame the null hypothesis in the "null" form such that there is no difference between the population parameters. Let Se_1 equal the true population sensitivity for imaging with Agent A and Se_0 equal the true population sensitivity with Agent B. Then, our statistical hypotheses for testing a difference between these sensitivities are

$$H_0 : Se_1 = Se_0$$

$$H_A : Se_1 \neq Se_0.$$

Note that the alternative hypothesis is two sided, meaning that the sensitivity of CT with Agent A could be either greater than or less than the sensitivity of CT with Agent B. We then collect study data and test whether the observed difference in the sensitivities we estimate from our study sample is unlikely to be due to chance. If this difference is large enough such that it would be unlikely to observe such a value (or something more extreme) if there were truly no differences in the population parameters, then we reject the null hypothesis in support of the alternative hypothesis. Note that if the p-value is not less than the prespecified significance level, then the evidence is insufficient to reject the null hypothesis. This does not mean we accept the null hypothesis of no difference.

8.3.3.2 Test for superiority

Sometimes we only care if a new imaging modality is better than the standard modality. If the new modality is not better or if it is worse, then we would not continue investigations of this modality. In this case, we state our alternative hypothesis such that the new test is better than the old. This is a one-sided test, as opposed to the two-sided test for a difference. For example, if we are interested in the sensitivity of the new (Se_1) versus standard (Se_0) modality, the hypotheses would be

$$H_0: Se_1 = Se_0$$
$$H_A: Se_1 > Se_0.$$

In this case, we would only reject the null hypothesis if Se_1 is sufficiently larger than Se_0 such that a difference of that magnitude (or larger) is unlikely to be observed if there were truly no difference. Note that we can only set up our alternative hypothesis in this way if we truly do not care if the sensitivity of the new modality is actually worse than the standard modality. With this setup, it is impossible to detect whether the new modality performs poorer. This situation is rare and will require defending.

8.3.3.3 Test for equivalence

In some cases, we want to show that a new imaging modality is as good as the standard modality. Say, there is an effective standard modality currently used in clinical practice. We developed a new modality we believe is as effective as the standard but with fewer side effects, less radiation exposure, lower cost, or greater convenience. We want to prove our new modality is as effective as the standard modality. When the hypothesis test is set up to detect a difference, failure to reject null hypothesis does not prove that the two modalities are equal. Thus, in the standard hypothesis testing setting for detecting differences, you can only conclude that the evidence is inadequate to show they are unequal. If the goal is to show the two modalities are equal, the study must be set up as an equivalency trial and the hypothesis test needs to be designed to demonstrate equivalence of the two modalities.

In equivalency trials, the null and alternative hypotheses are opposite of difference trials. However, it is impossible to demonstrate complete equivalency (i.e., no difference). Thus, we set up the hypothesis test based on a **margin of equivalence**, *M*, also called the **equivalence** or **tolerance limit**, which is the amount by which the two modalities would not be considered meaningfully different [11, 12]. Let Se_1 be the sensitivity of the new (experimental) modality and Se_0 be the sensitivity of the standard (old) modality. The null hypothesis is that the difference is outside the margin of equivalence, either the sensitivity of the new modality is better than the sensitivity of the standard modality by more than *M* or the sensitivity of the new modality is worse than the sensitivity of the standard modality by more than M:

$$H_0 : Se_1 - Se_0 \leq -M \quad \text{or} \quad Se_1 - Se_0 \geq M.$$

The alternative hypothesis is that the difference between the sensitivities of the new and standard modality is within the margin of equivalence, M, that is, that neither the new nor standard modality has a sensitivity that is better by more than M:

$$H_A : -M < Se_1 - Se_0 < M.$$

Figure 8.7 illustrates the margin of equivalence. If the probability that the difference $(Se_1 - Se_0)$ is outside this zone is less than 0.05, then we reject the null hypothesis and state that the new modality is equivalent to the standard modality. This is equivalent to the 95% confidence interval around the difference being completely within this zone, that is, if both the upper and lower confidence limits are within this zone (see Figure 8.7, Case A).

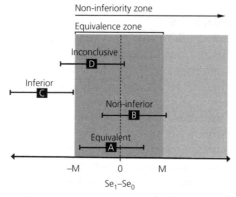

Figure 8.7 Illustration of tests of equivalence and noninferiority. Each line represents a 95% confidence interval. $Se_1 - Se_0$ is the difference in sensitivity of the new versus standard modality. For equivalence tests, if the confidence interval around the difference lies fully within the equivalence margins ($-M$ to M, dark shading), then we reject the null hypothesis and state that the new modality is equivalent to the standard modality (Case A). For noninferiority tests, if the lower confidence limit is larger than the noninferiority margin, $-M$ (i.e., the confidence interval is fully within the dark and light shading), we reject the null hypothesis and state that the test is not inferior (Case B); if the upper confidence limit is smaller than the noninferiority margin, we state that the test is inferior (Case C); and if the lower confidence limit is smaller than the noninferiority margin but the upper confidence limit is greater than the noninferiority margin, we cannot reject the null hypothesis, and the result is inconclusive (Case D).

8.3.3.4 Test for noninferiority

In some situations, we want to show that a new modality is at least as good as the standard modality, but we are not necessarily interested in whether it is superior. Similar to an equivalency trial, we set up the hypothesis test based on a **noninferiority margin**, M, which is the amount by which our new modality would not be considered meaningfully worse than the standard modality [11, 12]. Figure 8.7 illustrates the noninferiority margin. Let Se_1 be the sensitivity of the new (experimental) modality and Se_0 be the sensitivity of the standard (old) modality. The null hypothesis is that the sensitivity of the new modality is worse than the sensitivity of the standard modality by more than M:

$$H_0: Se_1 - Se_0 \leq -M.$$

The alternative hypothesis is that the difference between the sensitivities of the new and standard modality is larger than $-M$:

$$H_A: -M < Se_1 - Se_0.$$

We reject the null hypothesis and state that the new modality is not inferior to the standard modality if the lower confidence limit for the difference in sensitivities is larger than the noninferiority margin (see Figure 8.7, Case B). If the upper confidence limit is smaller than the noninferiority margin, we state that the test is inferior (see Figure 8.7, Case C). If the lower confidence limit is smaller than the noninferiority margin but the upper confidence limit is greater than the noninferiority margin, we cannot reject the null hypothesis, and the result is inconclusive (see Figure 8.7, Case D). Chapter 7 illustrates how to calculate sample size for testing noninferiority for Case example 1.1.

8.4 More on *p*-values

8.4.1 Problems with *p*-values

The p-value is the calculated probability of a test statistic differing the observed amount or more from the null hypothesis value by chance alone (under the null hypothesis model). Thus, the p-value tells you the **statistical significance** of your finding. The **practical significance**, or **clinical significance**, though, depends on the setting and the clinical and translational impact of your result (see Chapter 7 for discussion of an example illustrating these concepts).

8.4.2 Relationship between *p*-values and confidence intervals

For many, but not all, statistical procedures, there is a reciprocal relationship between the 95% confidence interval and the corresponding two-sided hypothesis test at the 0.05 significance level. For example, if we are interested in testing whether two means are significantly different, we could create a 95% confidence interval for the difference in the means. If the null hypothesis value (in this case, zero) is included in the 95% confidence interval, then the two-sided test at level 0.05 will not reject the null hypothesis. If the null hypothesis value is not included in the 95% confidence interval, then the two-sided test will reject the null hypothesis at 0.05. For our example of comparing the sensitivity of an imaging modality with and without a contrast agent, our null hypothesis is that the sensitivities are equal, which is equivalent to stating that the difference between the sensitivities is equal to zero. Thus, if the 95% confidence interval around the difference in the sensitivities excludes zero, we can reject the null hypothesis of no difference at the 0.05 level. If it includes zero, then the sensitivities are not significantly different. In contrast, it is important to point out that one cannot assume that if two sets of confidence overlap, the values are not significantly different. This is a common mistake made by researchers. The reciprocal relationship between confidence intervals and hypothesis tests is only true for a single confidence interval that directly corresponds to the hypothesis test of interest.

For one-sided hypothesis tests, the 0.05 significance level is all in one direction. A reciprocal relationship also exists between confidence intervals and corresponding one-sided hypothesis tests, but because we have 0.05 all in one direction, a 90% confidence interval must be used. If the lower limit of the 90% confidence interval excludes zero, then we can reject the null hypothesis.

In addition to reporting a *p*-value, a confidence interval should be provided, because it gives information on precision that is not provided by the *p*-value.

8.5 Advanced topics: statistical modeling

In this section we discuss statistical modeling in imaging studies. Although this is a more advanced mathematical topic, modeling is used extensively in imaging studies. We use statistical modeling to (i) compare two modalities when the subjects undergoing the two modalities are different and were not randomized (unpaired design—see Chapter 7), (ii) test if an outcome differs for subjects with different characteristics, (iii) predict outcome from imaging results, and (iv) reduce noise in the data. In this section we review the basic types of models and how the model parameters are interpreted.

All models have three basic parts: independent variable(s), dependent variable(s), and the mathematical function that links them. **Independent variables** are the predictors or variables that you need to adjust for. For example, in a study to assess if F-FDG predicts breast cancer mortality, age and cancer stage would be obvious independent variables that would need to be accounted for in predicting mortality. **Dependent variables** are the outcome variables. For imaging studies these might be the test result (positive or negative), a patient-reported functional or pain score, or the number of days until a subject's disease progresses or they die. We discuss modeling for three types of mathematical functions commonly used in imaging: linear, logistic, and time-to-event. The type of mathematical function depends on the type of dependent variable. If the dependent variable is a continuous variable, for example, tumor volume, then linear regression is used. If the dependent variable is binary, for example, positive or negative test result, then logistic regression is used. If the dependent variable is the time until an event, for example, time until progression, then we use a time-to-event model. We discuss the first two model types in this chapter; time-to-event models are discussed in Chapter 10.

8.5.1 Linear regression

A linear regression model takes the form $Y_i = \beta_o + \beta_1 X_1 + \beta_2 X_2 + \epsilon_i$, where Y_i is the outcome for the ith subject, β_o is the overall mean, X_1 and X_2 are the values of independent variables, β_1 and β_2, are the regression coefficients that we are interested in, and ϵ_i is the random error. Suppose that we want to determine if tumor volume (measured in mm³) is different for subjects undergoing two treatments and we want to control for the subject's age. We denote the treatments as $X_1 = 1$ for treatment A and $X_2 = 0$ for treatment B. We denote the subject's age as X_2. After controlling for the subject's age, we are interested in whether the treatment has any effect on tumor volume; in other words, whether the regression coefficient, β_1, is different from zero. There are several statistical methods to estimate β_1 and test if it differs significantly from zero; interested readers should consult standard textbooks such as Kutner et al. [13] for further details. Suppose that our estimate of β_1 is 2.5. We interpret this as follows: subjects undergoing treatment A have a mean tumor volume 2.5 mm³ larger than subjects undergoing treatment B.

8.5.2 Logistic regression

Suppose we want to identify factors that affect the sensitivity of the new liver blood-pool agent for detecting colorectal metastases at CT (Case example 1.1). We want to consider several potential predictors: the size of the lesion (categorized as <10 mm or ≥10 mm), the location of the lesion in the liver, and whether or not the subject has other comorbidities of the liver. We fit a model similar to the linear model in Section 8.5.1; however, since our dependent variable is binary (true positive or false negative), the mathematical function is a logit. The model takes the form $\ln \dfrac{F(x)}{1 - F(x)} = \beta_o + \beta_1 X_1 + \beta_2 X_2 + \beta_3 X_3$, where ln is the natural logarithm and $F(x)$ is the probability that the outcome is a success, for example, a true positive. In our example, X_1 might be the size of the lesion (0 if small, 1 if large), X_2 the location in the liver, and X_3 the presence/absence of comorbidities. Readers interested in the mathematics behind estimating the regression coefficients should see Hosmer and Lemeshow [14].

Now suppose that our estimate of β_1 is 1.25. To interpret this, we must transform it into an **odds ratio** using the formula e^{β_1}. We obtain an odds ratio of 3.5. Note that an odds ratio of 1.0 means that lesion size has no effect on the probability that the lesion is detected (i.e., no effect on sensitivity). We interpret our odds ratio of 3.5 as follows: after adjusting for effects due to the location of the lesion and comorbidities, the odds of a TP relative to an FN increase by 3.5 for large lesions. Note that the *sensitivity* is not 3.5 times greater for large lesions; rather, the *odds* of a TP relative to an FN are 3.5 times greater for large lesions. For example, suppose that our study sample includes 50 lesions: 27 small and 23 large. Among the small lesions, there are 12 TPs (sensitivity of 12/27 = 44%), and among the large lesions, there are 17 TPs (sensitivity of 17/23 = 74%). The odds of a TP:FN for large and small lesions are 17:6 and 12:15, respectively. The odds ratio is (17/6)/(12/15) = 2.83/0.80 or 3.5. The odd of a TP relative to an FN for large lesions (2.83) is 3.5 times larger than the odds of a TP relative to an FN for small lesions (0.8).

References

1 Sonnad, S.S., Describing data: statistical and graphical methods. *Radiology*, 2002. **225**(3): p. 622–628.
2 Remer, E.M., et al., Detection of urolithiasis: comparison of 100% tube exposure images reconstructed with filtered back projection and 50% tube exposure images reconstructed with sinogram-affirmed iterative reconstruction. *Radiology*, 2014. **272**(3): p. 749–756.
3 Sistrom, C.L. and C.W. Garvan, Proportions, odds, and risk. *Radiology*, 2004. **230**(1): p. 12–19.
4 Medina, L.S. and D. Zurakowski, Measurement variability and confidence intervals in medicine: why should radiologists care? *Radiology*, 2003. **226**(2): p. 297–301.
5 Brown, L., T. Cai, and A. DasGupta, Interval estimation for a binomial proportion. *Stat Sci*, 2001. **16**: p. 101–133.
6 Tufte E., *The Visual Display of Quantitative Information*. 2001, Graphics Press: Cheshire, CT.
7 Blume, J. and J.F. Peipert, What your statistician never told you about *P*-values. *J Am Assoc Gynecol Laparosc*, 2003. **10**(4): p. 439–444.
8 Tello, R. and P.E. Crewson, Hypothesis testing II: means. *Radiology*, 2003. **227**(1): p. 1–4.
9 Zou, K.H., et al., Hypothesis testing I: proportions. *Radiology*, 2003. **226**(3): p. 609–613.
10 Applegate, K.E., R. Tello, and J. Ying, Hypothesis testing III: counts and medians. *Radiology*, 2003. **228**(3): p. 603–608.
11 Piaggio, G., et al., Reporting of noninferiority and equivalence randomized trials: extension of the CONSORT 2010 statement. *JAMA*, 2012. **308**(24): p. 2594–2604.
12 Walker, E. and A.S. Nowacki, Understanding equivalence and noninferiority testing. *J Gen Intern Med*, 2011. **26**(2): p. 192–196.
13 Kutner, M., C. Nachtsheim, and J. Neter, *Applied Linear Regression Models, 4th ed*. Operations and Decisions Sciences. 2004, McGraw Hill/Irwin: Boston, MA.
14 Hosmer, D., S. Lemeshow, and R. Sturidivant, *Applied Logistic Regression, 3rd ed*. 2013, John Wiley & Sons, Inc.: New York.

CHAPTER 9

Methods for studies of diagnostic tests

Jeffrey D. Blume

Vanderbilt University, Nashville, TN, USA

KEY POINTS

- The uncertainty in data is comprised of systematic variation and random variation. Random variation is controlled through the sample size, while systematic variation is controlled through the design or with post hoc statistical methods (e.g., stratification or regression analysis).

- Kappa statistics measure agreement for categorical data, while intraclass correlation coefficients (ICCs) measure agreement for continuous data.

- There is a natural trade-off between sensitivity and specificity. Accurately characterizing that trade-off is the goal of summarizing diagnostic test performance. Reporting only a single sensitivity/specificity pair is not best practice and should be avoided.

- The accuracy of a diagnostic test is represented by a receiver operating characteristic (ROC) curve, which plots a test's sensitivity versus 1-specificity for every possible operating point.

- The area under an ROC curve (AUC) is a summary measure of test's diagnostic ability. In complex study designs with multiple readers, the average AUC is used as summary measure (but it is far from perfect).

9.1 Introduction

This chapter introduces statistical methods commonly used in studies of diagnostic tests. Typically the goal is to assess the degree to which different diagnostic tests agree or to measure the accuracy of a particular test. Some methods are straightforward, such as when the study design features only a single test, but some are complex, such as when the study design features multiple modalities (i.e., multiple tests) and multiple readers (i.e., multiple test interpreters).

Handbook for Clinical Trials of Imaging and Image-Guided Interventions, First Edition.
Edited by Nancy A. Obuchowski and G. Scott Gazelle.
© 2016 John Wiley & Sons, Inc. Published 2016 by John Wiley & Sons, Inc.

In general, the statistical approach is this: select and compute a summary statistic, calculate its variability, and report the point estimate and its confidence interval (CI). The CI, typically set at a 95% level, provides the range of values that are consistent with the data, and this range is compared against clinically meaningful benchmarks. If the CI contains only clinically meaningful or only clinically irrelevant effect sizes, then the study is said to generate strong, possibly definitive, evidence. If the CI contains both meaningful and nonmeaningful effect sizes, then the study is said to be inconclusive and to yield only weak evidence.

This chapter is organized as follows: we first discuss sources of statistical and scientific variation, so that they may be controlled experimentally (if at all possible). If experimental control is not possible, then statistical methods of control—stratification or regression adjustment—can be used. Of course, statistical control can be complicated, and it is often less desirable than experimental control. Next is a discussion of how to measure agreement among multiple tests. We then introduce the concept of diagnostic accuracy and explain how it can be measured. In closing, we touch on elements of generalizability and an advanced regression technique (logistic regression) that is useful in this arena.

9.2 Sources of variation

Perhaps the defining feature of a rigorous and well-controlled study is that potential sources of variation are identified in the planning stage and controlled through experimental conditions. For example, radiologist performance is impacted by experience, training, and routine. Variation among radiologists in these criteria will almost surely lead to increased variation in the outcome data and subsequent reduction in power and precision. The goal, of course, is to minimize the extent of statistical variability, which can be envisioned as having two components: a random part (sometimes called the natural variability or variation due to unknown factors) and a systematic part (sometimes called the variability due to experimental conditions or variation due to knowable factors). Increasing the sample size reduces random variation. Systematic variation, on the other hand, cannot be controlled in this way. If the source of variation can be identified, it can be controlled either by experimental means or by statistical means (stratification or regression analysis) post hoc.

Impactful factors can either be controlled (e.g., only "experienced" radiologists are used as readers) or balanced (e.g., an equal number of "experienced" and "inexperienced" radiologists are readers). Controlling these factors limits the generalizability of the study, but it also substantially reduces variation and thus increases statistical power. Balancing factors increases generalizability, but then special statistical techniques (e.g., regression methods) are needed to properly account for and attribute the observed sources of variation [1]. Clearly, there is a balancing act here. However, it is always much better to deal with these issues up front, as statistical adjustments may not always achieve the desired results.

We will assume that studies are well controlled so that regression adjustments of key summary measures are not needed. This avoids much mathematical complexity and allows us to focus on the concepts. But the reality is that it is not possible to experimentally control every source of variation and regression methods are almost always needed.

9.3 Assessing the agreement among multiple tests

It is often of interest to know whether two (or more) different tests or readers agree in their assessment of a particular image, assay, or participant. Importantly, agreement does not imply "correctness" or "accuracy"; it is possible to have perfect agreement without any accuracy whatsoever. Thus, agreement endpoints should be carefully considered in the context of any diagnostic evaluation.

The simplest of these designs collects the assessments of each reader on every image. If there are n images to be assessed and r evaluators, the study generates r columns of n assessments, with a row for each image. There are various metrics of agreement for two evaluators, depending on the type of outcome being assessed (e.g., categorical or continuous). Extensions to multiple evaluators typically involve computing all pairwise agreements metrics and then averaging them. Here we introduce the two most common metrics of agreement: the kappa statistic for categorical outcome data and the intraclass correlation coefficient (ICC) for continuous outcome data.

9.3.1 Categorical data and the kappa statistics

For categorical outcome data, such as dichotomous or ordinal outcomes, a **kappa statistic** is used to assess agreement [2]. It is helpful to imagine the tabulated data when there are only two readers evaluating a set of images. Such a table would have one reader's scores in columns and the other reader's scores along the rows (see Table 9.1 and associated discussion for an example with two tests). Each image is put into the cell that corresponds to its evaluations. The diagonal elements of the table indicate agreement, and the sum of all diagonal elements equals the total number of images on which the two readers (or two tests) agree. This type of tabulation works only because the outcome data—the reader scores—are categorical.

The kappa statistic is essentially the percent agreement "corrected" (i.e., reduced) for accidental or chance agreement. As a result of this correction, the range of a kappa statistic is from -1 to 1. Kappas less than 0.4 indicate poor agreement, kappas between 0.4 and 0.75 indicate fair to good agreement, and kappas greater than 0.75 indicate excellent agreement [2]. Altman [4] suggests a more refined scale: less than 0.2 (poor), 0.2 to 0.4 (fair), 0.4 to 0.6 (moderate), 0.6 to 0.8 (good), and greater than 0.8 (very good). There are two extensions of kappa statistics worth mentioning.

Table 9.1 Example of kappa statistics.

All participants with complete data Kappa is 0.44 95% CI (0.41, 0.47)		Integrated test results		
		+	–	Total
Mammography	+	107	29	141
Test results	–	199	2302	2571
	Total	306	2331	2637
Positive reference standard Kappa is 0.35 95% CI (0.09, 0.61)		Integrated test results		
		+	–	Total
Mammography	+	19	1	20
Test results	–	12	8	20
	Total	31	9	40
Negative reference standard Kappa is 0.41 95% CI (0.38, 0.45)		Integrated test results		
		+	–	Total
Mammography	+	88	28	116
Test results	–	187	2294	2481
	Total	275	2322	2597

Source: Data and table adapted from an American College of Radiology Imaging Network (ACRIN) study of combined ultrasound and mammography screening versus mammography screening alone in women at high risk for breast cancer. Adapted from Berg, et al. [3].

The first common extension allows kappa statistics to give partial credit for "near" agreements. These modified kappa statistics are called **weighted kappa statistics**. Near agreements are off-diagonal elements "close" to the main diagonal. For example, if the outcome scale is from 1 to 10, the cell for score pairs (5,6) and (6,5) might be considered a "near" agreement. The manner in which score pairs are weighted varies, and the weighting scheme has a large impact on the resulting magnitude of the weighted kappa. Accordingly, the weights should be decided before any data are collected, or else it is tempting to be more generous in defining near agreement after the fact.

The second common extension is the **multireader kappa**, which is used as a measure of overall agreement when there are more than two evaluators. In these situations, it is always a good idea to report the observed range of kappa statistics that arise from all pairings. If there are r raters, then the number of pairing is $\binom{r}{2} = \dfrac{r!}{(r-2)!2!}$ where $r! = r(r-1)(r-2)\cdots1$ is the factorial operation. This number grows quickly; so simply presenting all pairwise kappas is often not feasible. Instead, the distribution of pairwise kappas is described, perhaps with a boxplot or simple quantiles. An average kappa is reported as the overall measure of agreement for the group of evaluators. In fact, a **multireader kappa** is just a weighted average of the pairwise kappas [2]. The weights can be constant, yielding a straight average, or they can reflect the proportion of data used for each pairwise kappa [2]. A similar procedure is used for weighted kappas, producing a multireader weighted kappa (i.e., a weighted average of weighted pairwise kappas). Weighted kappas and multireader kappas are interpreted on the same scale as kappa statistics (see discussed above).

Hypothesis tests and significance tests of kappa statistics and their extensions should be avoided [1]. Best practice is to report those levels of agreement that are best supported by the data, as given by a CI (see Chapter 8 for a discussion of CIs). If the interval is sufficiently narrow, then the data are to be interpreted as evidence for a particular level of agreement. If the CI is wide, then the data are said to be inconclusive. By default, most statistical software packages report the p-value from a significance test of the null hypothesis that the agreement is zero. However, these automatic tests are virtually meaningless. Why? Because they lack any consideration of clinical significance (which is already hard to characterize on the kappa scale) and they mask imprecision in small sample sizes. For example, the test of agreement might reject the null hypothesis that the agreement is exactly zero, but the CI might extend from 0.05 to 0.7 (indicating the data are effectively inconclusive with regard to agreement) or from 0.01 to 0.1 (indicating there is virtually no agreement).

9.3.2 Example: kappa statistics

The American College of Radiology Imaging Network (ACRIN) conducted a study of combined ultrasound and mammography screening versus mammography screening alone [3]. This is an example of a study design where two different "tests" are used to evaluate a participant. The study was conducted in 2809 women who had elevated risk of breast cancer. Although 2712 participants underwent with both screens, only 2637 yielded reference standard information (40 were positive, 2597 were negative).

Screening results from the integrated read (combined ultrasound and mammography) and from mammography alone were dichotomized as a positive or negative. Details can be found in Berg et al. [3]. These data are shown in Table 9.1, along with the kappa statistic that measures agreement between the integrated test and mammography alone. 95% CIs are also reported. Disease status is an important factor, so results are stratified by reference standard.

Here the overall kappa is 0.44 with a 95% CI ranging from 0.41 to 0.47. This indicates poor to fair agreement, with almost 10% (=228/2331) of participants on the off diagonals. Agreement stratified by reference standard shows consistent results, indicating the tests are no more or less likely to agree when the woman has cancer than when she does not. Notice that the overall kappa (0.44) is greater than either stratified kappa (0.35, 0.41). This implies that agreement is slightly better overall than in either of the reference standard groups, which, when combined, yield the larger group. This is somewhat unintuitive, and it happens because the correction for chance agreement is sensitive to how the data are

Table 9.2 Example of multireader kappa statistics.

Parameter	Multirater kappa (range of pairwise kappas)		p-value (null hypothesis is no agreement)	
	CT	MR imaging	CT	MR imaging
Tumor visualization	0.16 (0.12 to 0.29)	0.32 (0.22 to 0.41)	$p < 0.001$	$p < 0.001$
Invasion of right parametrium	−0.04 (−0.02 to 0.13)	0.10 (0.06 to 0.27)	$p = 0.961$	$p < 0.001$
Invasion of left parametrium	−0.05 (−0.01 to 0.11)	0.12 (0.05 to 0.29)	$p = 0.981$	$p < 0.001$
Staging	0.26 (0.23 to 0.34)	0.44 (0.34 to 0.56)	$p < 0.001$	$p < 0.001$

Source: Data from a retrospective study of CT and MR imaging for early invasive cervical cancer. Adapted from Hricak et al. [5].

combined. The take-home message is that kappa statistics will not necessarily behave as one might expect, and caution is warranted when examining agreement within subgroups.

An example of the use of multireader kappas is found in the report of an ACRIN/GOG study of early invasive cervical cancer [5]. The study examined the evaluation of 146 cases on CT by 4 readers and 152 cases on MR by 4 readers. Table 9.2 is adapted from the paper. It shows multireader kappa values along with the range of all pairwise kappas and p-values for testing the null hypothesis of no agreement (i.e., testing that the true kappa is zero).

Inclusion of 95% CIs would have strengthened the presentation, but the ranges do permit an assessment of the clinical relevance. Despite the significant p-values, agreement is quite poor. This is an excellent example of why statistical significance should not be mistaken for clinical importance. For example, in 5 out of the 6 instances where the p-value is highly significant, the observed range of multirater kappas clearly indicates poor agreement (i.e., the pairwise kappas are never more than 0.41). Agreement for MR staging was the highest, but even then the observed agreement appears moderate at best.

9.3.3 Continuous data and the ICC

Continuous outcome data, such as tumor volume or standardized uptake value (SUV), cannot be concisely tabulated. When the underlying measurements are continuous, it is nontrivial to define exactly what constitutes agreement because two measurements can be very close yet still not equal. So, for these types of data, the metric of agreement is the **ICC**, which measures agreement on the scale of variability (or "reliability" in the sense of less variance means more reliable). The idea is that measurements that are nearly identical can be considered reliable if their differences account for only a small fraction of the overall variability in the outcome measurement. That is, repeated measurements on a single case are considered reliable if the measurement differences tend to be small relative to differences from case to case.

Agreement for pairs of tests can be depicted with a **Bland–Altman plot** [6, 7]. Instead of plotting the two test outcomes versus one another, Bland–Altman plots display the difference in outcomes versus their average (so-called difference vs. mean plots). This allows visualization of potentially systematic problems, such as when the discrepancy in outcome measures increases as the outcome's magnitude increases. For further discussion of this useful tool, see Bland and Altman [6, 7] and reference therein. It is not uncommon for Bland–Altman plots to be presented without reference to an ICC; the visual depiction of agreement is often more informative that its single number summary.

9.3.4 Example: Bland–Altman plots

For illustration, consider Case example 1.1 from Chapter 1. The goal is to evaluate the diagnostic accuracy of a new liver blood-pool agent for detecting colorectal metastases on CT imaging. Call the new agent "A-new" and the current standard of care "B-old." We will assume both agents yield a continuous score derived from the CT image and/or its interpretation. Figure 9.1 displays the Bland–Altman plot for 40 simulated CT scores from each agent (paired by image). Overall there does

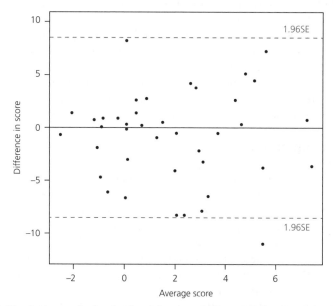

Figure 9.1 Bland–Altman plot for simulated data from 40 images under Case example 1.1. The y-axis is the difference in agents CT scores (A-new minus B-old) for detecting colorectal metastases. Dashed lines indicate ± 1.96 standard errors on the difference in scores.

not seem to be any concerning patterns; there is perhaps one outlier. The red dashed lines show the two standard error bands; agreement tends to be within ± 8.5 units. The next step would be to consider whether this level of agreement (±8.5 units) is clinically meaningfully.

For a published example of Bland–Altman plots, see the study on pulmonary nodules by Gietema et al. [8]. In this study 20 patients were twice scanned with low-dose CT. The main conclusion that "variation of semiautomated volume measurements of pulmonary nodules can be substantial" was supported with a Bland–Altman plot [8].

The **ICC** is the proportion of total outcome variance due to cases or images. Thus, $1 - \text{ICC}$ is the proportion of total variance due to reader disagreement. ICCs are always positive and cannot be greater than 1. As such, the scale of agreement is as follows: ICCs less than 0.4 indicate poor reliability, ICCs between 0.4 and 0.6 indicate fair reliability, ICCs between 0.6 and 0.75 indicate good reliability, ICCs between 0.75 and 0.85 indicate excellent reliability, and ICC greater than 0.85 indicate near perfect reliability [9–11]. When the contribution to the overall variance from reader disagreement is small, the ICC will be near one.

It is often helpful to examine each source's contribution to the overall variability. The attribution of variance to a single source is called a variance component (the components must sum to the total observed variance). ICCs are general enough to handle multiple readers, but they depend on an underlying statistical model for which the proper construction and estimation is nontrivial. The construction of the underlying model is beyond the scope of this chapter. Interested readers are referred to [11] and [10].

For ICCs as well, it is best to avoid hypothesis and significance testing. The variance due to a single source, or the ICC itself, is almost never exactly zero. Rather, the relevant question is, "How large is the reader variance?" or "How reliable are the tests?" Hence, best practice is to report the estimated levels of agreement that are best supported by the data. That is, one should report a CI for the ICC and any variance components of interest. An example is helpful to fix ideas.

9.3.5 Example: ICC

A modern example of the usage of ICCs and variance components to assess agreement between tests is found in an ACRIN study of two semiautomated systems for computing the volume of brain tumors from MR images of patients with new postoperative and recurrent malignant gliomas [13]. The study was a retrospective reader study, consisting of 16 readers (staff, fellows, and technologists) and 24 cases. Three platforms used to measure tumor volumes: 3DViewnix, Eigentool, and manual measurements. Tumor volume assessments were completed on each platform for Gd-enhancing and FLAIR hyperintensity lesions. The ICCs and variance components are shown in Table 9.3.

The data tell an interesting story. With FLAIR hyperintensity, we see that for 3DViewnix 95% of the variability in tumor measurements is due to case variation. In contrast, only 35% of the variability in Eigentool tumor measurements is due

Table 9.3 Example of intraclass correlation coefficients (ICC) and variance components.

		FLAIR hyperintensity		Gd-enhancing	
		Variance component	ICC (95% CI)	Variance component	ICC (95% CI)
3D Viewnix-TV	Cases	2,009.08	0.95 (0.92, 0.98)	89.09	0.51 (0.40,0.71)
	Readers	0.00	0.00 (0.00, 0.01)	0.00	0.00 (0.00,0.06)
	Error	102.82	0.05 (0.02, 0.07)	87.05	0.49 (0.28,0.59)
	Total	2,111.89	—	176.12	—
Eigentool	Cases	226.53	0.35 (0.26, 0.57)	76.84	0.25 (0.12,0.53)
	Readers	1.66	0.00 (0.00, 0.1)	0.00	0.00 (0.00,0.09)
	Error	422.40	0.65 (0.42,0.69)	232.64	0.75 (0.44,0.85)
	Total	650.60	—	309.47	—
Manual	Cases	2,782.05	0.44 (0.33, 0.61)	397.98	0.18 (0.14,0.39)
	Readers	0.00	0.00 (0.00, 0.06)	0.00	0.00 (0.00,0.10)
	Error	3,564.82	0.56 (0.37,0.66)	1,825.26	0.82 (0.58,0.84)
	Total	6,346.87	—	2,223.23	—

Source: Data from a reader study of software platforms for computing volume changes over time in participants with malignant gliomas. Adapted from Ertl-Wagner et al. [13].

to case variation, much like manual measurement (44%). Interestingly enough, in all cases, variability across readers is virtually nonexistent.

Conclusions drawn from ICCs, however, can be misleading. This is because the overall magnitude of variability is masked by the ICC. The units associated with variance are volume squared. Notice that 3DViewnix-TV reduces the variability in FLAIR volume measurements by a factor of 3, while Eigentool reduces it by a factor of 10. The problem is that ICCs explain proportional reduction, not absolute reduction. Eigentool has less proportional reduction (i.e., most of the variability cannot be attributed to cases nor readers). Nevertheless, Eigentool has substantially less variability—it is more reliable overall—when measuring FLAIR volumes. For Gd-enhancing lesions, the two software platforms are essentially equivalent (an easy way to see this is that the ICC for 3DViewnix-TV, 51%, is within the 95% CI of Eigentool's ICC, so their performance is not statistically different). The degree to which the two software platforms yield similar tumor volume measurements for any given case is also addressed in the paper [13].

9.4 Assessing the accuracy of diagnostic tests

When evaluating a diagnostic test, a more rigorous standard than agreement is test performance. Namely, how often does the test correctly identify a diseased or nondiseased subject? It turns out that this seemingly simple question has a complicated answer. Why? Because the answer depends on how the test is used in practice. A single test can appear to have multiple performance profiles, so a sophisticated metric is needed to properly summarize it.

A helpful analogy is the breaking distance of a car (i.e., the distance, in feet, that a car takes to come to a complete stop). Clearly, the breaking distance of a car depends on how fast the car is moving; faster cars take longer to come to a complete stop. As such, it makes little sense to compare the breaking distances of two cars traveling at different speeds. The distances are not comparable (there is no reason to expect them to be the same); in statistical language we say that the breaking distance of a car is confounded by speed. In order to compare breaking distances, we need to "control" for speed. We might do this in several ways. The simplest approach is to hold speed constant and only compare breaking distances at the same speed, say, breaking distance at 60 MPH. A more complex approach is to display, and visually compare, the breaking distance *curves* (breaking distance on the *y*-axis vs. speed on the *x*-axis). While the curve comparison is clearly more informative (it shows the simplest approach at every speed), it is hard to summarize in a single number. It turns out that summarizing a test's diagnostic performance has this same problem.

9.4.1 Notation

In order to assess test performance, we need to know the test score and the true underlying disease state of the subject being tested. The latter is formally known as the reference standard (gold standard is an outdated term), which we will represent as D_i for the ith participant's disease status. So $D_i = 1$ if the ith participant has the disease and $D_i = 0$ if not. For n participants, the total number of diseased participants is $n_d = \sum_{i=1}^{n} D_i$, and the number of nondiseased subjects is $n_n = \sum_{i=1}^{n} (1 - D_i)$. Clearly, $n = n_d + n_n$.

The simplest of study designs collects the test score and reference standard on each of n participants. That is, it collects the pairs (X_i, D_i), where X_i is the ith participant's test score. If there are t tests under investigation, the data collected is $(X_{1i}, ..., X_{ti}, D_i)$, and the study generates $t + 1$ columns of data with n rows each. The complexity in defining and collecting reference standard information is discussed elsewhere, but it should not be overlooked. Poor reference standard ascertainment will doom even the best of studies.

9.4.2 Test performance: Sensitivity and specificity

The **sensitivity** of a test measures how often the test correctly indicates that a subject is diseased. The **specificity** measures how often the test correctly indicates that a subject is not diseased. The caveat is that tests, by themselves, provide only a score, not an indication. For that, we need a benchmark, or cutoff, that we can compare the test score against. Then if the test score, X_i, is greater than the cutoff, say c, we will say the test indicates that the subject has the disease or that the subject "tested positive." The indicator function, $I(X_i > c)$, allows us to compactly write down this process: $I(X_i > c) = 1$ if $X_i > c$ and $I(X_i > c) = 0$ if $X_i \le c$.

Table 9.4 The typical 2×2 table of diagnostic outcomes.

Cutpoint = c	Diseased	Nondiseased	Total
Test positive	TP(c)	FP(c)	n_+
Test negative	FN(c)	TN(c)	n_-
Total	n_d	n_n	n

The definitions of diagnostic test results, when using a specific cutoff, are illustrated.

The computation formulae for sensitivity and specificity, at a given cutpoint c, are

$$\mathrm{Sens}(c) = \frac{\mathrm{TP}(c)}{n_d} = \frac{\sum_{i=1}^{n} I(X_i > c) D_i}{\sum_{i=1}^{n} D_i}$$

$$\mathrm{Spec}(c) = \frac{\mathrm{TN}(c)}{n_n} = \frac{\sum_{i=1}^{n} (1 - I(X_i > c))(1 - D_i)}{\sum_{i=1}^{n} (1 - D_i)}$$

where TP(c) is the number of diseased participants with scores greater than c (the "true positives") and TN(c) is the number of nondiseased subjects with scores less than c (the "true negatives"). Also, we will use FN(c) for the number of diseased participants with scores less than c (the "false negatives") and FP(c) for the number of nondiseased subjects with scores greater than c (the "false positives"). The summary table of test performance, based on cutpoint c, is shown in Table 9.4.

It is critically important to remember that this table changes as the cutpoint c changes. As the test is used differently, its performance profile changes. This means that a reported sensitivity (or specificity) for two different tests cannot be compared without careful thought. Just as in the braking distance example, the comparison of sensitivity (or specificity) across tests is almost surely confounded. One solution to this problem is to hold the cutpoint constant within any comparison. However, different tests tend to have different outcome scales (and hence different cutpoint scales), so holding the cutpoint constant is not always an option. In these situations, we typically hold one performance measure constant while comparing the other. For example, we might compare the sensitivities of two tests at whatever cutpoint makes their specificity equal.

It is important to remember that sensitivity and specificity are fundamentally connected, so that comparisons of one performance measure, without regard to the other, are largely misdirected. For the same reason attempting to maximize sensitivity or maximize specificity, without regard to the other, is meaningless. Imagine a broken test that simply indicated every patient was diseased. This test has sensitivity of 100%, but its specificity is zero. There is a natural trade-off between sensitivity and specificity. Accurately characterizing that trade-off is the goal of summarizing diagnostic test performance.

9.4.3 Test performance: positive predictive value and negative predictive value

The **positive predictive value (PPV)** measures how often the subject is really diseased when the test yields a positive result. The **negative predictive value (NPV)** measures how often the subject is not diseased when the test is negative. PPV and NPV are the clinically meaningful quantities that are used in assessing the clinical value of a test result for an individual patient. The computation formulae for PPV and NPV, at a given cutpoint c, can also be seen from Table 9.4 as

$$\text{PPV}(c) = \frac{\text{TP}(c)}{n_+} = \frac{\sum_{i=1}^{n} I(X_i > c) D_i}{\sum_{i=1}^{n} I(X_i > c)}$$

$$\text{NPV}(c) = \frac{\text{TN}(c)}{n_-} = \frac{\sum_{i=1}^{n} (1 - I(X_i > c))(1 - D_i)}{\sum_{i=1}^{n} (1 - I(X_i > c))}$$

The formulae are similar to that for sensitivity and specificity, except that the denominators have now changed to the number of participants who tested positive $n_+ = \sum_{i=1}^{n} I(X_i > c)$ and the number of participants who tested negative $n_- = \sum_{i=1}^{n} (1 - I(X_i > c))$, with cutpoint c. From an experimental perspective this change is significant because the denominators can no longer be controlled by design. As a result, the prevalence of disease in the sample directly influences $\text{PPV}(c)$ and $\text{NPV}(c)$, introducing another source of variation to account for.

Studies of diagnostic tests are typically designed and analyzed in sensitivity/specificity space because these measures are not influenced by the prevalence and because the classical experimental paradigm is that of examining how well the test works under known conditions (i.e., when the disease status is already known). Moreover, if PPV and NPV are of interest, which they often are, then they can be readily computed after the fact. It turns out that $\text{PPV}(c)$ and $\text{NPV}(c)$ are functionally related to $\text{Sens}(c)$ and $\text{Spec}(c)$ via a specific formula that is given by Bayes' theorem (see Chapter 10). Thus, $\text{PPV}(c)$ and $\text{NPV}(c)$ can always be computed from $\text{Sens}(c)$ and $\text{Spec}(c)$ if the disease prevalence is known. Figure 9.2 displays this relationship for $(\text{Sens}(c), \text{Spec}(c))$ pairs of $(0.9, 0.9)$, $(0.5, 0.5)$, and $(0.25, 0.25)$.

Bayes' theorem is used often in practice. However, there is a school of thought that advocates for directly estimating PPV and NPV without first estimating sensitivity and specificity [14–17]. While useful in some contexts, this approach has not become mainstream.

9.4.4 Receiver operating characteristic curves and the area under the curve

A car's stopping distance profile is given by its breaking distance curve (breaking distance on the y-axis vs. speed on the x-axis). Although the curve is not easy to summarize with a single number, inspecting it can be quite informative (especially

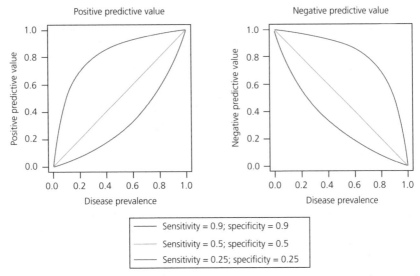

Figure 9.2 Positive predicted value (PPV) and negative predicted value (NPV) as a function of sensitivity, specificity, and disease prevalence.

since cars tend to be driven at different speeds). The same principle is true for diagnostic tests.

A test's performance prolife is also represented by a curve; a single sensitivity/specificity pair is insufficient to describe how the test might perform in practice. The curve that describes a test's performance profile is called a **receiver operating characteristic (ROC) curve**. The ROC curve plots sensitivity (on the y-axis) versus 1-specificity (on the x-axis) for all possible cutpoints c. In our notation, the plot consists of the points $(1 - \text{Spec}(c), \text{Sens}(c))$ for every possible c; each point corresponding to a tabulation like that given by Table 9.4.

Figure 9.3 displays two example ROC plots. The left panel shows four different operating points, or cutpoints, on a single ROC curve. The right panel shows the same four operating points, but here each comes from its own ROC curve. The point is that when we only observe four operating points, the assumption that they all come from a single ROC curve is a strong one. For example, even if the data for all four operating points comes from the same clinical site, it could be that the test is being used slightly differently in each case (and hence their underlying ROC curves are truly different). The solution to this problem is to avoid inference based on a single operating point. That is, collect the test score instead of the determination if the test is positive or negative. Then estimate and present the entire ROC curve. Get out of the habit of thinking about a test's diagnostic performance in terms of a single sensitivity/specificity pair.

It is unusual, but not unheard of, to plot sensitivity (or specificity) versus the cutpoint. The reason for this is a practical one: not all tests have cutpoints on the same scale, so multiple curves cannot always be drawn on the same graph. Plotting

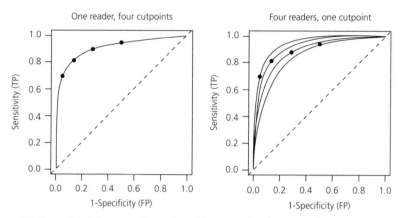

Figure 9.3 Example ROC curves. Illustration of four cutpoints from a single ROC curve versus four cutpoints from four different ROC curves. The four points on each graph are identical, illustrating the danger in assuming only a single curve exists.

sensitivity versus 1-specificity resolves this problem and provides a more compact display. A note on naming conventions: sensitivity is the true positive fraction (TPF) and 1-specificifty the false positive fraction (FPF), so the ROC curve is a plot of the TPF versus the FPF.

Inspecting the ROC curve is always informative, and it would be helpful if it were possible to summarize, with a single number, the trade-off between sensitivity and specificity that is displayed by the ROC curve. While no single metric is perfect for this task [18, 19], the **area under the curve (AUC)** is the current standard for doing this. The AUC can be estimated in a variety of different ways and is often referred to as the **diagnostic accuracy** of the test. The most common approach is to use the trapezoidal rule to approximate the AUC. This estimator is nonparametric (i.e., it makes few statistical assumptions) and also unbiased [12, 20, 21]. There are other approaches, such as parametric or model-based estimates, kernel smoothing estimators, or simple numerical integration.

The classic nonparametric estimate of the AUC is

$$\widehat{AUC} = \frac{\sum_{i=1}^{n_d}\sum_{j=1}^{n_n} I\left(Y_i^D > Y_j^{\bar{D}}\right) + I\left(Y_i^D = Y_j^{\bar{D}}\right)/2}{n_d n_n}$$

where $Y_1^D,...,Y_{n_d}^D$ are the test scores of diseased subjects and $Y_1^{\bar{D}},...,Y_{n_n}^{\bar{D}}$ are the test scores of nondiseased subjects. Here $I\left(Y_i^D = Y_j^{\bar{D}}\right) = 1$ if $Y_i^D = Y_j^{\bar{D}}$ and 0 otherwise. This empirical estimate of the AUC is also known as the Mann–Whitney U-statistic [12, 20]. The formula for its variance can be found in Zhou et al. [20], Pepe [21], and Hanley and McNeil [12]. $\widehat{AUC}$ estimates the true area under the ROC curve, which is

$$AUC = P\left(Y^D > Y^{\bar{D}}\right).$$

That is, the AUC has a nice interpretation as the probability that a randomly selected test score from a diseased subject, Y^D, will be greater than a randomly selected test score from a nondiseased subject, $Y^{\bar{D}}$. [12]. The AUC measures the tendency for diseased test outcomes to be larger than nondiseased test outcomes. An AUC of one means the test always yields higher scores for diseased subjects, and AUC of ½ means there is no inherent ordering (i.e., the test does not discriminate). Unfortunately, the AUC can be insensitive to important but small changes in the shape of the ROC curve [22]. Other summaries are available, for example, the partial AUC, but they have not been widely adopted. See Pepe [21] for examples.

9.4.5 Example: illustration of ROC curves

Let's return to the simulated data for Case example 1.1 from Chapter 1. The goal here is to evaluate the diagnostic accuracy of a new liver blood-pool agent for detecting colorectal metastases on CT imaging. The new agent is called "A-new" and the standard of care is called "B-old." We would like to compare the agents in terms of their ability to detect liver metastases based on CT imaging.

Figure 9.4 displays boxplots and the ROC curves of observed CT scores. The two figures are complementary. The boxplots show the empirical distributions of CT scores for the new agent and old agent. For each agent, the empirical ROC and its smooth ROC curve (assuming a binormal model (Metz, Herman, Shen [23])) are displayed. Notice that for agent A-new, the boxplots for disease and nondiseased scores have more separation (i.e., less overlap). This implies that A-new CT scores are a slightly better discriminator for disease status. The ROC plots show this reality more clearly; the ROC curve for A-new dominates the curve for B-old. This means that at any specificity, A-new will operate with a higher sensitivity.

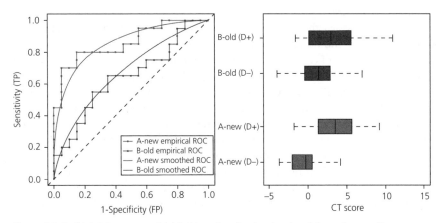

Figure 9.4 (Left) ROC curves and (right) boxplots for the simulated data of a new liver blood-pool agent from Case example 1.1. Data from 40 simulated participants: 20 disease positive and 20 disease negative. For boxplots the solid black line is the median; whiskers extend to the observation closest to the fence without exceeding it. Top ROC curve corresponds to "A-new," bottom ROC curve corresponds to "B-old."

Table 9.5 AUC statistics for simulated liver metastases example in Case example 1.1.

	Agent		
	A-new	**B-old**	**p-value**
Empirical AUC (95% CI)	0.86 (0.74, 0.98)	0.64 (0.47, 0.82)	0.0412
Smoothed AUC (95% CI)	0.87 (0.76, 0.98)	0.66 (0.50, 0.83)	0.0496

Statistics computed using R v3.1 and STATA v12.1.

Table 9.5 shows the empirical and smoothed AUCs and their 95% CIs. It also gives the p-value for testing that the two areas are the same. In both cases, the data suggest that the AUC for A-new is higher than B-old at the 5% level (albeit barely). With only 40 cases, an apparently large improvement in discrimination ability of the new agent is almost washed out by insufficient precision.

9.5 Multireader multimodality studies

It is often the case that a diagnostic test does not produce an objective quantitative score. The most common examples of this are imaging tests where a physician or technologist must read, or interpret, an image. Because different readers may interpret images differently, the diagnostic accuracy of the "test" depends on the reader. In an ideal setting, the image would be clear enough that all readers would have the same interpretation, but this does not always happen. Because of this, it is important to assess the degree to which reader variation affects the diagnostic accuracy of the test.

In order to assess the effect of reader variation on the diagnostic accuracy of the test, a study should have many different readers read the same set of cases under the same set of conditions. Statistical methods [20] for analyzing these data are complex and varied, but there are a number of important points that are worth mentioning. First, the data should not be pooled over readers. The general principle for analysis is that each reader's diagnostic accuracy/performance should be estimated first, and then accuracy across readers is estimated from those reader-specific summaries. This order is important because pooling reader data amounts to assuming that everyone is operating similarly with respect to cut-points, and this is often not the case. Second, reader characteristics that would affect interpretation should be controlled or balanced. Third, a broad case spectrum should be used whenever possible to provide a generalizable assessment of performance.

Multireader studies typically involve multiple readers interpreting common set of imaging studies derived from one or more diagnostic abilities. A well-controlled multireader study has a uniform imaging protocol, a common set of cases that all readers of evaluate, and a common procedure for ascertaining the reference standard of each case. A variety of complex analytical approaches are available [20]. Most methods require dedicated effort from a statistician familiar with these techniques.

9.5.1 Example: reader study of computer-aided diagnostic for breast MR interpretation

Lehman et al. [22] report results from a reader study designed to compare the diagnostic accuracy of breast MR imaging interpretation with and without a computer-aided diagnostic (CAD) system in novice and expert readers. The study recruited 20 readers to evaluate 70 different cases twice: once with CAD and once without. Of the 20 readers, 9 were experts and 11 novices. Of the 70 cases, 27 were benign and 43 were malignant. The order of the readings was randomly determined for each reader, and rereads of cases were separated by 6 months to inhibit recall bias.

Readers recorded their interpretation of the breast MR in three different ways, each a different outcome scale designed to record the reader's intuitive probability that the lesion was malignant. The three outcome scales were (i) the BI-RADS scale without the zero category, (ii) a 5-point probability malignancy scale (normal, probably normal, equivocal, probably abnormal, definitely abnormal), and (iii) the readers' actual estimate of the chance that the lesion was malignant (on a continuous scale from 0 to 100, called percent probability of malignancy). These data permit an assessment of the relative utility of these scales. While Lehman et al. [22] observed minor variation in the overall assessment of accuracy across the three scales, there are some statistical reasons for preferring scales with more categories.

Table 9.6 shows the average AUC, with and without CAD, on each scale. We see that CAD appears to improve diagnostic accuracy by a small amount.

Table 9.6 Example of a multireader multimodality study.

	Outcome scale	Average AUC With CAD	Without CAD	p-value
All (20 readers)	BI-RADS	0.8091	0.7841	0.0890
	Probability of malignancy scale	0.8191	0.7917	0.0865
	Percent probability of malignancy	0.8238	0.8036	0.2529
Experienced	BI-RADS	0.8266	0.7972	0.1308
(9 readers)	Probability of malignancy	0.8383	0.8058	0.0752
	Percent probability of malignancy	0.8431	0.8231	0.1941
Novice	BI-RADS	0.7949	0.7734	0.2665
(11 readers)	Probability of malignancy	0.8033	0.7801	0.2390
	Percent probability of malignancy	0.8080	0.7876	0.3881

Source: Data from a reader study of a computer-aided diagnostic (CAD) system to aid breast MR interpretation. Data adapted from Lehman et al. [22].
Table displays the average AUC with and without CAD on three different outcome scales.

Table 9.7 Example of a multireader multimodality study.

	Reader ID	CAD (modality 1)		No-CAD (modality 2)		p-value
		AUC	Standard error	AUC	Standard error	
Novice readers	1	0.8586	0.0411	0.8039	0.0500	0.2062
	2	0.8771	0.0475	0.7967	0.0489	0.1231
	3	0.8405	0.0445	0.8274	0.0468	0.7929
	4	0.7761	0.0567	0.7471	0.0575	0.6399
	5	0.8577	0.0444	0.7963	0.0557	0.2588
	6	0.7765	0.0559	0.6763	0.0656	0.123
	7	0.8119	0.0558	0.8396	0.0513	0.4504
	8	0.7757	0.0577	0.7984	0.0561	0.6596
	9	0.7281	0.0588	0.7862	0.0537	0.2734
	10	0.7866	0.0568	0.7458	0.0591	0.4677
	11	0.7479	0.0606	0.7639	0.0567	0.831
Experienced readers	12	0.8493	0.0501	0.8077	0.0486	0.2715
	13	0.7416	0.0601	0.7921	0.0532	0.4056
	14	0.8809	0.0434	0.8245	0.0460	0.2128
	15	0.8434	0.0502	0.8068	0.0512	0.5048
	16	0.8636	0.0412	0.7942	0.0511	0.1472
	17	0.8346	0.0534	0.8253	0.0505	0.8443
	18	0.8733	0.0433	0.7997	0.0553	0.0446
	19	0.8632	0.0449	0.8136	0.0529	0.0969
	20	0.7946	0.0587	0.7879	0.0599	0.8289
	Average	0.8191		0.7917		0.0865

Source: Data from a reader study of a computer-aided diagnostic (CAD) system to aid breast MR interpretation. Data adapted from Lehman et al. [22].
Table displays each reader's AUC with and without CAD on the probability of malignancy outcome scale.

Experienced readers showed a slightly higher accuracy than novice readers overall, but here too the increase in average accuracy was small (2–4 percentage points in the AUC). For these data, there does not appear to be a reason to prefer one outcome scale over another. It is reassuring to see the same general patterns across different scales, with experienced readers performing slightly better than novices and CAD having a slight advantage over No-CAD. Of note, the p-values in this table are computed from a carefully specified ANOVA model that accounts for reader-to-reader variability, the details of which are complex [24].

To understand where the average AUCs in Table 9.6 come from, consider Table 9.7, which shows the reader-specific AUCs, with and without CAD, on the probability of malignancy scale.

The reader-specific AUCs are the empirical or nonparametric estimators. Here the standard error for each AUC is shown, and the within reader p-value for testing no change in AUC is reported. Notice that only reader 18 shows a statistically

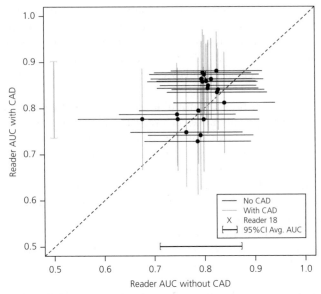

Figure 9.5 Display of reader-specific AUCs in the CAD MR reader study. 95% CIs for each AUC are the points. The vertical lines are CIs for the group when using CAD. The horizontal lines are CIs for group when not using CAD. The CI for the average AUC (over all readers) is plotted along the axis for that group. Reader 18 is the second most top-left point. Source: Data from Lehman [22].

significant improvement, at the 5% level, in accuracy due to CAD. The 95% CI for the average CAD accuracy is 0.7367–0.9014, and the CI for average accuracy without CAD is 0.7108–0.8726. More importantly, the 95% CI on the difference in average accuracy was −0.0043–0.0591. This interval includes zero and values near zero, which helps explain the marginal p-value of 0.0865.

The degree of variability exhibited by the data is hard to glean from Table 9.7. However, Figure 9.5 shows it clearly.

Each reader's AUC pair (without CAD, with CAD) is plotted as a single point. The red lines show the 95% CI for the CAD AUC, while the blue lines show the 95% CIs for the without CAD AUC. The 95% CI for the average AUC over all readers is plotted near the axis and bracketed for reference. Unfortunately, the point cloud is quite close to the dashed line of agreement. While only five points are below the line of agreement, the points above remain close to the line. When the variability of the points is considered, it becomes clear that these data do not strongly support a hypothesis of large accuracy improvement due to CAD.

Lehman et al. [22] report on other important differences in operational sensitivity, PPV, NPV and the average time to complete reads, which are not discussed here. Reader-specific ROC curves are also displayed in Lehman et al. [22], but in this case the AUCs tell most of the story. One important finding is that the extent of reader variation observed in this study was nontrivial. For an example of a reader study that exhibited low variability between readers, see the ACRIN study of MR spectroscopy for prostate cancer localization [25]. Lastly, note the precision in the CAD study that resulted from using 20 readers and 70 cases. The precision on the estimated AUC difference was 2–3 percentage points, quite small when comparing AUCs and certainly well within the limits of a clinical meaningful change in AUC.

Lastly, a cautionary note about multicenter studies of diagnostic tests is that multireader studies typically have each reader interpret every case. This design increases power, allows the experimenter to identify the degree of reader-to-reader variability, and uses each case as its own control. However, it can be tempting for a center to use a group of readers to handle a reading load. When this happens, the effect is that each center represents an amalgamation of various interpreters. This should be avoided whenever possible. The added variability from assuming that a group of readers can be just as consistent as a single reader can greatly increase statistical variance and reduce power. In addition, the observed accuracy for the group will be an attenuated estimate of the ideal accuracy.

9.5.2 A note on combining ROC curves or their AUCs

An important issue is how to actually obtain an average ROC curve over multiple readers. Like with kappa statistics, how we average is important. We know to avoid averaging over different operating points, but how does one average an entire ROC curves? The answer is model dependent, unfortunately. There are several ways to define an average ROC curve. For example, one could average curves vertically (by specificity) or horizontally (by sensitivity). Alternatively, if the curves can be parameterized, it might be possible to average the parameters that govern the curve's shape rather than the curves themselves. The problem, of course, is that the average AUC would not then be equal to the AUC from the model with average parameters. That is, the average ROC curve has an area that is not equal to the average ROC area. This happens because the averaging spaces are nonlinear, so the decision of where to average, in terms of averaging curves or averaging areas, is an important choice. One widely accepted practice is that of averaging the nonparametric estimates of the AUC, as we did in the previous example.

9.5.3 Elements of generalizability

The generalizability of a study comes directly from the design of the study. The reader population, for example, may be expert readers or professionals at large from the community. The performance of an academic expert would not be expected to represent well the performance of professionals at large. Expert readers may provide the upper ceiling of accuracy for a technology, but they tend not to well represent the expected performance at large. Similarly, nonexpert readers provide valuable feedback about what is achievable for professionals at large and how effective training can be in practice.

Case spectrum is another important aspect of study design that requires careful thought. Ideally, it is best to have a representative sample of all forms of disease. A more uniform case sample might reduce variability in performance criteria, but it also reduces the generalizing of the results to everyday practice. It is also possible that the sample prevalence may influence reader's interpretation, and for this reason the sample prevalence is often kept from the readers so as to not change their reading behavior.

The design of the study with respect to reader and case generalizability is just as important as outlining the technical characteristic of the imaging process. The studies generalize to phenomena that they mimic well. If a certain factor is not included in the study in sufficient numbers, then the study does not generalize well to that factor. Readers and cases are obvious example, but other important factors are reading conditions, resource pressures, machine type, software, and imaging parameters. More on study design and generalizability can be found in Zhou, Obuchowski, and McClish [20].

9.6 Logistic regression as tool for obtaining AUCs

One particularly useful tool for evaluating diagnostic test data is logistic regression. As we learned in Chapter 8, logistic regression is a statistical model for the probability of disease, which is allowed to depend on predictors. Predictors can be test scores or demographic variables. In fact, a logistic regression with only a single predictor will yield the nonparametric estimate of the AUC for that predictor (in regression terminology the AUC is known as the c-statistic). What is useful about this technique is that other factors can be added to the model to force balance or to compare tests, albeit with some limitations [26]. The model can identify a factor's impact on the diagnostic accuracy of a test, and it can also adjust for redundant information from several different tests.

A logistic regression yields a **risk score** based on the included predictors. This risk score is essentially a new diagnostic test, and the accuracy of the risk score for predicting disease status is given by its AUC or c-statistic. Some software packages provide a CI for the c-statistic, but most do not. A simple solution is to use bootstrapping techniques, if available. Another reason to employ a logistic regression model is that they can handle missing data via multiple imputation. A detailed discussion is beyond the scope of this chapter, but regression methods are a powerful tool for advanced analysis of diagnostic test data.

References

1 Blume, J. and J.F. Peipert, What your statistician never told you about *P*-values. *J Am Assoc Gynecol Laparosc*, 2003. **10**(4): p. 439–444.
2 Fleiss, J.L., Measuring nominal scale agreement among many raters. *Psychol Bull*, 1971. **76**(5): p. 378–382.

3 Berg, W.A., et al., Combined screening with ultrasound and mammography vs mammography alone in women at elevated risk of breast cancer. *JAMA*, 2008. **299**(18): p. 2151–2163.

4 Altman, D.G., *Practical Statistics for Medical Research*. 1991, Chapman and Hall: London.

5 Hricak, H., et al., Early invasive cervical cancer: CT and MR imaging in preoperative evaluation—ACRIN/GOG comparative study of diagnostic performance and interobserver variability. *Radiology*, 2007. **245**(2): p. 491–498.

6 Bland, J.M. and D.G. Altman, Statistical methods for assessing agreement between two methods of clinical measurement. *Lancet*, 1986. **1**(8476): p. 307–310.

7 Bland, J.M. and D.G. Altman, Measuring agreement in method comparison studies. *Stat Methods Med Res*, 1999. **8**(2): p. 135–160.

8 Gietema, H.A., et al., Pulmonary nodules: interscan variability of semiautomated volume measurements with multisection CT—influence of inspiration level, nodule size, and segmentation performance. *Radiology*, 2007. **245**(3): p. 888–894.

9 Koch, G., Interclass correlation coefficient, in *Encyclopedia of Statistical Sciences 4*, S. Kotz and N. Johnson, Editors. 1982, John Wiley & Sons, Inc.: New York. p. 213–217.

10 Donner, A. and J.J. Koval, The estimation of intraclass correlation in the analysis of family data. *Biometrics*, 1980. **36**(1): p. 19–25.

11 Shrout, P.E. and J.L. Fleiss, Intraclass correlations: uses in assessing rater reliability. *Psychol Bull*, 1979. **86**(2): p. 420–428.

12 Hanley, J.A. and B.J. McNeil, The meaning and use of the area under a receiver operating characteristic (ROC) curve. *Radiology*, 1982. **143**(1): p. 29–36.

13 Ertl-Wagner, B.B., et al., Reliability of tumor volume estimation from MR images in patients with malignant glioma. Results from the American College of Radiology Imaging Network (ACRIN) 6662 Trial. *Eur Radiol*, 2009. **19**(3): p. 599–609.

14 Harrell, F., *Regression Modeling Strategies*. 2001, Springer: New York.

15 Cook, N.R., Statistical evaluation of prognostic versus diagnostic models: beyond the ROC curve. *Clin Chem*, 2008. **54**(1): p. 17–23.

16 Moons, K.G., et al., Limitations of sensitivity, specificity, likelihood ratio, and bayes' theorem in assessing diagnostic probabilities: a clinical example. *Epidemiology*, 1997. **8**(1): p. 12–17.

17 Moons, K.G.M. and F.E. Harrell, Sensitivity and specificity should be de-emphasized in diagnostic accuracy studies. *Acad Radiol*, 2003. **10**(6): p. 670–672.

18 Hand, D., Measuring classifier performance: a coherent alternative to the area under the ROC curve. *Mach Learn*, 2009. **77**(1): p. 103–123.

19 Hand, D.J. and C. Anagnostopoulos, When is the area under the receiver operating characteristic curve an appropriate measure of classifier performance? *Pattern Recogn Lett*, 2013. **34**(5): p. 492–495.

20 Zhou, X., N.A. Obuchowski, and D.K. McClish, *Statistical Methods in Diagnostic Medicine, 2nd ed.* 2011, John Wiley & Sons, Inc.: Hoboken, NJ.

21 Pepe, M.S., *The Statistical Evaluation of Medical Tests for Classification and Prediction*. Oxford Statistical Science Series. 2004, Oxford University Press: Oxford.

22 Lehman, C.D., et al., Accuracy and interpretation time of computer-aided detection among novice and experienced breast MRI readers. *AJR Am J Roentgenol*, 2013. **200**(6): p. 683–689.

23 Metz, C.E., B.A. Herman, and J.H. Shen, Maximum likelihood estimation of receiver operating characteristic (ROC) curves from continuously-distributed data. *Stat Med*, 1998. **17**(9): p. 1033–1053.

24 Obuchowski, N.A. and H.E. Rockette, Hypothesis testing of diagnostic accuracy for multiple readers and multiple tests: an ANOVA approach with dependent observations. *Commun Stat Simul Comput*, 1995. **24**: p. 285–308.

25 Weinreb, J.C., et al., Prostate cancer: sextant localization at MR imaging and MR spectroscopic imaging before prostatectomy—results of ACRIN prospective multi-institutional clinicopathologic study. *Radiology*, 2009. **251**(1): p. 122–133.

26 Pepe, M.S., et al., Limitations of the odds ratio in gauging the performance of a diagnostic, prognostic, or screening marker. *Am J Epidemiol*, 2004. **159**(9): p. 882–890.

CHAPTER 10

Methods for quantitative imaging biomarker studies

Alicia Y. Toledano[1] and Nancy A. Obuchowski[2]

[1] Biostatistics Consulting, LLC, Kensington, MD, USA
[2] Quantitative Health Sciences, Cleveland Clinic Foundation, Cleveland, OH, USA

KEY POINTS

- A quantitative imaging biomarker (QIB) is "an objective characteristic derived from an in vivo image measured on a ratio or interval scale as indicators of normal biological processes, pathogenic processes or a response to a therapeutic intervention."

- Bias and precision are key components to describing the technical performance of a quantitative imaging system.

- Repeatability and reproducibility are different measures of precision. Repeatability describes the variability in a subject's measurements, holding all imaging procedures constant. Reproducibility describes variability in a subject's measurements when at least one imaging procedure (e.g., scanner, reader, institution) is changing. Both measures are needed to fully characterize an imaging system's precision.

- LoB, LoD, LoQ, linearity, and commutability are important analytic properties of QIBs.

10.1 Quantitative imaging biomarkers

Many of the numbers that arise from clinical examinations can be considered biomarkers. They provide information about health at the time of measurement and may also provide information about future health risks. The term **biomarker** is formally defined by the US Food and Drug Administration (FDA) as "a characteristic that is objectively measured and evaluated as an indicator of normal biological processes, pathogenic processes, or pharmacologic responses to a therapeutic intervention" [1]. The National Institutes of Health (NIH) Biomarkers Definitions Working Group uses a similar definition [2].

Medical images are increasingly acquired in digital, rather than analog, format. This allows for advanced image processing and facilitates attaching

Handbook for Clinical Trials of Imaging and Image-Guided Interventions, First Edition.
Edited by Nancy A. Obuchowski and G. Scott Gazelle.
© 2016 John Wiley & Sons, Inc. Published 2016 by John Wiley & Sons, Inc.

numbers to image properties. Such **quantitative imaging** is formally defined by the Radiological Society of North America (RSNA) as "the extraction of quantifiable features from medical images for the assessment of normal or the severity, degree of change, or status of a disease, injury, or chronic condition relative to normal. Quantitative imaging includes the development, standardization, and optimization of anatomical, functional, and molecular imaging acquisition protocols, data analyses, display methods, and reporting structures. These features permit the validation of accurately and precisely obtained image-derived metrics with anatomically and physiologically relevant parameters, including treatment response and outcome, and the use of such metrics in research and patient care" [3]. These extracted features are considered **quantitative imaging biomarkers (QIBs)**. One of the RSNA's Quantitative Imaging Biomarkers Alliance (QIBA) working groups recently published consistent terminology surrounding QIBs [4]. The group defines a QIB as "an objective characteristic derived from an in vivo image measured on a ratio or interval scale as indicators of normal biological processes, pathogenic processes or a response to a therapeutic intervention."

Measurement on an interval scale ensures that the difference between two values is meaningful. Consider, for example, tumor volume in cubic centimeters (cm^3): a $2\,cm^3$ change in tumor volume is the same change whether it is from 2 to $4\,cm^3$ or from 20 to $22\,cm^3$. The clinical implications may differ, but the absolute difference has the same meaning.

This is not true for ordinal data, that is, data on a numerical scale for which order matters but spacing between numbers is not equal. For example, consider the Breast Imaging Reporting and Data System (BI-RADS) assessment categories: the two-category difference between a BI-RADS category 1 (negative) and a BI-RADS category 3 (probably benign) does not have the same meaning as the two-category difference between a BI-RADS category 3 and a BI-RADS category 5 (highly suggestive of malignancy) [5]. In the first instance, the woman whose mammograms received a category 1 assessment has "essentially 0% likelihood of malignancy," and the recommended management is routine screening mammography, whereas the woman whose mammogram received a category 3 assessment has greater than 0% but at most 2% likelihood of malignancy, and the recommended management is short-interval follow-up or continued surveillance mammography. At most the increase in likelihood of malignancy is 2%, and the change in management is an earlier visit focusing on the lesion leading to the category 3 assessment. In the second instance the woman whose mammogram received a category 5 assessment has at least 95% likelihood of malignancy, and the recommended management is tissue diagnosis. Here a 2-category difference is associated with at least a 93% increase in likelihood of malignancy and an invasive procedure. Ordinal scales such as the BI-RADS assessment categories play important roles in medical care; this example serves merely to illustrate that they are not part of the set of what would be considered QIBs.

While measurement on an interval scale ensures that the difference between two values is meaningful, measurement on a ratio scale goes a step further: it ensures that the ratio of two values also is meaningful. Ratio variables must have a unique, not arbitrary, zero value. Tumor volume in cubic centimeters has this ratio scale property: a change from 2 to 4 cm³ is a doubling of tumor volume, as is a change from 20 to 40 cm³; zero volume means that there is no measured tumor. Although not an imaging biomarker, a familiar example of an interval scale that does not have the ratio scale property is temperature. An interval of 5°F measures the same change in temperature whether it is from 50 to 55°F or 75 to 80°F. The difference between temperature and tumor volume is that 0°F does not correspond with absence of temperature, so 80°F is not twice as hot as 40°F.

10.2 Evaluating the technical performance of QIBs

In order to determine the applicability and validity of a QIB, it is crucial that the framework in which they are acquired is well described including the context of use, acquisition parameters, measurement methodology, and quantification of performance. Knowledge of these factors enables clinicians to reliably compare measurements over time and across imaging platforms [4]. In this section we discuss methods for quantifying the technical performance of a quantitative imaging procedure.

10.2.1 Bias

The quantity that the QIB intends to measure is called the **measurand**. Suppose we perform a phantom study to assess the technical performance of a new CT software system for measuring the volume of lung tumors. The QIB is tumor volume in cubic centimeters as measured by CT using a specified acquisition protocol and specified measurement protocol, and the measurand is the actual tumor volume in the subject at the time of measurement. **Bias** is the difference between the average of the measurements and the measurand.

Suppose in our example we take five measurements on each of 10 synthetic lesions (see Table 10.1). Let Y_{ik} denote the kth measurement on the ith lesion. To estimate bias, we first compute the mean of the five measurements for each lesion; we denote this $\bar{Y}_i$ for the ith lesion. Thus, $\bar{Y}_i = \sum_{k=1}^{K}(Y_{ik})/K$, where K is the total number of measurements taken for each lesion, that is, $K=5$ in our example. From Table 10.1, the mean of the measurements for the first tumor is 0.482. Let X_i denote the true volume of the ith lesion ($X_i = 0.5$ for the first tumor). The bias for lesion i is $(\bar{Y}_i - X_i)$. For lesion $i=1$ the estimated bias is −0.018. An estimate of the overall bias, that is, an average over all lesions, is $\sum_{i=1}^{N}(\bar{Y}_i - X_i)/N$, where N is the total number of lesions. In our example, $N=10$ and the estimated bias is −0.013, which means that our CT software tends to underestimate the true volume by 0.013 cm³. We would want to construct a 95% confidence interval for the bias as well (see Chapter 8 for a discussion of confidence intervals).

Table 10.1 Measured volumes (in cm³) of 10 hypothetical tumors.

Volume (cm³)	Measurement					Mean	Bias	% Bias	wSD$_i$
	1	2	3	4	5				
0.5	0.43	0.45	0.50	0.63	0.40	0.482	−0.018	−3.6	0.090
1.0	0.88	1.09	1.04	0.91	1.02	0.988	−0.012	−1.2	0.089
1.5	1.48	1.34	1.37	1.39	1.51	1.418	−0.082	−5.5	0.073
2.0	2.18	2.08	2.07	2.03	1.99	2.070	0.070	3.5	0.071
2.5	2.37	2.50	2.34	2.72	2.52	2.490	−0.010	−0.4	0.151
3.0	2.89	2.90	2.91	3.01	3.09	2.960	−0.040	−1.3	0.087
3.5	3.31	3.68	3.56	3.61	3.36	3.504	0.004	0.1	0.161
4.0	3.78	4.13	4.06	3.95	3.83	3.950	−0.050	−1.3	0.148
4.5	4.45	4.41	4.49	4.72	4.71	4.556	0.056	1.2	0.148
5.0	4.93	4.91	5.02	4.86	5.05	4.954	−0.046	−0.9	0.079

Overall bias = −0.013; wSD for all lesions = 0.11.
Repeatability coefficient = 2.77 × wSD = 0.304.

Investigators often report **percent bias**, which is the estimated bias divided by the true value times 100 [4]. This measure is used when it is believed that the magnitude of the bias depends on the magnitude of the true value. Note that percent bias can only be evaluated when the QIB has a meaningful zero (see Section 10.3.5).

10.2.2 Repeatability

The potential utility of a QIB can be greatly impacted by lack of **repeatability**, which is the consistency of results when the same QIB is assessed at short intervals on the same subject using the same equipment at the same imaging center. More formally, the **repeatability condition of measurement** is a "set of conditions that includes the *same* measurement procedure, *same* operators, *same* measuring system, *same* operating conditions and *same* physical location, and replicate measurements on the same or similar experimental units over a short period of time" [4].

Repeatability studies are sometimes called **test–retest studies**. In these studies, subjects are scanned once and then asked to return for a second scan in a period of time sufficiently short to allow no biologic change in the subject's condition (e.g., 15 min to several weeks, depending on the disease). Repeatability can also be assessed in phantom studies, but for some diseases a phantom may not be representative of the complexity of patients' disease, and thus repeatability may be underestimated in these studies [6].

The **within-subject standard deviation** (wSD) is a commonly used metric for describing repeatability. Using the example from Section 10.2.1, we first estimate the wSD for each lesion as follows: $\text{wSD}_i = \sqrt{\sum_{k=1}^{K}(Y_{ik} - \overline{Y}_i)^2 / (K-1)}$. For example, for the first lesion in Table 10.1, the $\text{wSD}_i = 0.090$. To get an estimate of wSD for all lesions, we take the mean of the wSD_i over the N lesions, $wSD = \sum_{i=1}^{N=10} wSD_i / N$. In the example in Table 10.1, the estimate of the wSD is 0.11.

The **repeatability coefficient** (RC) is defined as 2.77 times the wSD. The difference in any two measurements on the same subject is expected to be between −RC and +RC for 95% of subjects. This is why the RC is also sometimes called the 95% limits of agreement. The amount of repeatability required for a QIB to be useful depends on its intended use.

10.2.3 Reproducibility

The potential utility of a QIB can also be greatly impacted by lack of **reproducibility**, which is defined as consistency of results when the same QIB is assessed at short intervals on the same subjects using *different* equipment. This **reproducibility condition of measurement** is "a set of conditions that includes *different* locations, operators, measuring systems, and replicate measurements on the same or similar objects" [4]. Reproducibility studies require making multiple measurements on the same subject but with different scanners, with different imaging software, with different readers, or at different imaging centers. Note that not all of these conditions need to be met in a single study. For example, if the study design calls for imaging each subject with two different scanners at a single institution with one reader, then the reproducibility condition is met.

Reproducibility is often measured by the **intraclass correlation coefficient**, which is the proportion of total variance in the QIB values that is explained by the variance between scanners (or imaging centers and/or different readers, etc.). Different study designs lead to different formulae for the intraclass correlation coefficient depending on whether each subject is interpreted by the same set of readers, or by different readers, and on whether the readers are considered to be a sample from a larger population of potential readers. Perfect agreement leads to an intraclass correlation coefficient of one. Another commonly used measure of reproducibility is the **reproducibility coefficient** (RDC), which has an interpretation analogous to the RC in Section 10.2.2 [6].

Bland–Altman plots are often used to illustrate an imaging procedure's bias and precision. These plots are on the same scale as the QIB values and show the difference of measurements versus their average. The mean difference and mean difference plus or minus two SDs are often labeled; the latter are called the 95% **limits of agreement**. See Chapter 9 for an illustration.

Developing reproducible QIBs can be difficult. It is important to consider all of the possible sources of variability. For example, subject-related variability in QIB values can occur because of positioning or motion. Similarly, imaging system-related variability in QIB values can be related to procedures, operators, operating conditions, and/or software. The presence of these types of excess variability in QIB values can make measured changes in QIB values difficult to interpret [7].

10.3 Evaluating analytical properties of QIBs

10.3.1 Detection capability: limits of blank, detection, and quantification

Important clinical questions relate to small values: How small a tumor can we find? How accurate are volumes of small tumors? How do we know that something with a small volume is not an artifact? We can adapt principles for answering similar questions about *in vitro* diagnostic tests [8] to answering these questions about QIBs. In doing so, it will be important to retain as much information about small volumes as possible. For example, if a computer algorithm automatically displays values below $0.5\,cm^3$ as 0, we would want to either decrease that threshold or extract the calculated volume before it is rounded down.

We can assess whether something with a small volume is an artifact by comparing the volume with the **limit of the blank** (LoB). The LoB is the "threshold above which measurements from the quantity with true state of measurand = 0 are obtained with probability α (probability of falsely claiming that the true state of measurand > 0)." The value of α is usually 0.05. Conversely, we can assess whether something represents an actual tumor with the **limit of detection** (LoD). The LoD "is the measured quantity value, obtained by a given measurement procedure, for which the probability of falsely claiming that the true state of measurand = 0 is β, given a probability α of falsely claiming that the true state of measurand > 0." The value of β also is usually 0.05 [4].

One way to obtain an LoB and LoD for a particular CT acquisition protocol and tumor volume measurement procedure would be with anatomical phantoms containing designated regions without simulated lesions as well as simulated lesions of small, known volumes. The morphology of these simulated lesions might vary from spherical, to reflect lesion morphologies in a disease of interest. We would incorporate all of the factors that might influence measurements into our experiment, for example, multiple technicians, multiple measurers if humans perform this task, multiple days, and possibly multiple phantoms. The total number of measurements should be sufficient to provide some certainty in the results while not being overly burdensome; CLSI EP17-A2 suggests a minimum of 60 replicates for each "blank" (region without simulated tumor volume) and each "low-level sample" (small tumor volume) [8]. The simplest way to obtain the LoB is then to sort all of the blank measurements from lowest to highest; calculate the rank of the percentile corresponding to α; the LoB is that ranked measurement. If there are multiple blank regions of interest, we can obtain the LoB separately for each and then the overall LoB is the highest of them; or we can pool the measurements. Establishing the LoD is more complex; we use one of the several possible procedures in the following text.

Example

Consider using a phantom with two blank regions and six simulated small spherical lesions, two each with volumes 0.1, 0.2, and 0.3 cm³ (approximate diameters = 0.58, 0.73, and 1.79 cm), and obtaining 60 measurements on each. Set $\alpha = \beta = 0.05$. From one blank region we obtain in increasing order: 0, 0, ..., 0.0380 cm³, 0.0410 cm³, 0.0497 cm³, 0.0529 cm³; from the other: 0, 0, ..., 0.0383 cm³, 0.0393 cm³, 0.0453 cm³, 0.0541 cm³. For $\alpha = 0.05$ and 60 replicates we need the 57.5th ranked value, obtained as the average of the 57th and 58th ranked values. This is 0.0395 cm³ for the first blank region and 0.0388 cm³ for the second. We take the LoB as the higher of these, 0.0395 cm³. From our simulated small lesions, we obtain a pooled SD of 0.0268 cm³. We inflate this by a constant derived from β, the 360 total measurements, and the number of lesions and add it to the LoB to obtain LoD = 0.0836 cm³ [8] (see Figure 10.1). We can interpret these as measured volumes 0.0395 cm³ or less can be considered artifacts; actual tumor volumes as small as 0.0836 cm³ can be measured.

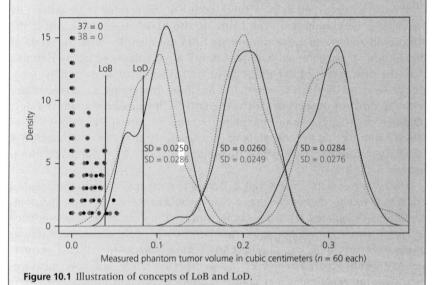

Figure 10.1 Illustration of concepts of LoB and LoD.

The **limit of quantitation** (LoQ) is "the lowest value of measurand that can be reliably detected and quantitatively determined with {stated} acceptable precision and {stated, acceptable} bias, under specified experimental conditions" [4]. The LoQ is based on goals related to clinical applications—for example, therapy decisions. Bias is a systematic measurement error, whereas repeatability and reproducibility are different measures of precision. Bias and precision goals for an LoQ may address each aspect separately or through a combined total error measure [4]. As with LoD, we again incorporate all of the factors that might influence measurements into our experiment; and the total number of measurements should be sufficient to provide some certainty in the results while not being overly burdensome. CLSI EP17-A2 suggests a minimum of 36 replicates for each potential LoQ under consideration [8]. This highlights an important distinction compared with LoB and LoD: we select trial values of the LoQ and determine whether measurement at each value occurs with "{stated} acceptable precision and {stated, acceptable} bias," rather than relying solely on the statistical properties of the measurement procedure.

Example, continued

The phantom tumor volumes are treated as known, such that bias can be measured separately from precision. We will use %RMS for root mean square (RMS) defined as the square root of the sum of bias squared and SD squared, as our combined measure of bias and precision. Our criterion is that the LoQ can be quantitatively determined with %RMS less than 20%. For the 0.1 cm^3 phantom lesions, we observed (mean = 0.1012, SD = 0.0250) and (mean = 0.0945, SD = 0.0286). Estimated bias is then 0.0012 and –0.0055 and %RMS = 25.0 and 29.1%. Neither of these meet the stated criterion, so we cannot claim LoQ = 0.1 cm^3. For the 0.2 cm^3 phantom lesions, we observed (mean = 0.2036, SD = 0.0260) and (mean = 0.2020, SD = 0.0249), such that %RMS = 13.1 and 12.5%. Both of these meet our stated criterion. The LoQ for tumor volume measured with this acquisition protocol, and this measurement procedure is then claimed as 0.2 cm^3.

10.3.2 Linearity and commutability

Linearity means that the QIB values have a linear relationship with the measurand. If the value of the measurand is X and the value of the QIB is Y, this means that $Y = a + bX$. An everyday example is temperature conversion from degrees Celsius to degrees Fahrenheit, with $a = 32°$ and $b = 1.8$: $°F = 32 + 1.8°C$. The $a = 32°$ is an offset to reflect that freezing, 0°C, happens at 32°F. Once that shift occurs, each °C is equal to 1.8°F. Thus boiling, 100°C, happens at $32° + 1.8 \times 100°C = 212°F$. A special case of linearity is **proportionality**, in which there is no offset $(a = 0)$.

As in the previous section, we can adapt principles for answering similar questions about *in vitro* diagnostic tests [9]. The approach examines whether a nonlinear polynomial fits data better than a linear one; if so, it assesses whether the difference between the best-fitting nonlinear and linear models is less than an amount of allowable bias. The experiment uses a series of known values in, or extending slightly beyond, a linear range of interest. The high end of the range should take into consideration medical decision limits within the clinical context. To establish a range, 9–11 known values are preferred, and each value should have at least two replicates. It is important that the phantom be similar to the organ in which the lesions are located. If this is not possible, healthy patient samples with inserted levels of the QIB may be required. It is also important to make the measurements in random order to prevent any carry-over effects.

Example, continued

We are interested in establishing linearity from a lower limit of the LoQ, $0.2\,\text{cm}^3$, through a maximum of $5\,\text{cm}^3$ (in a spherical lesion this corresponds with a $2.12\,\text{cm}$ diameter). We use the data in Table 10.2. Figure 10.2 shows the relationship between the measurand and the CT measurements. We then fit three regression models to the data: linear, curvilinear, and s shaped, to be sure. Results of those fits are shown in Table 10.3. The nonlinear terms in the s-shaped model are not statistically significant (p-value > 0.05), so we do not need both a Volume^2 and Volume^3 term. The nonlinear term in the curvilinear model also is not statistically significant, so we do not need a Volume^2 term. The linear model fits best, and we can say that tumor volume measured with this acquisition protocol and this measurement procedure is linear from $0.2\,\text{cm}^3$ through $5\,\text{cm}^3$.

Table 10.2 Hypothetical data for assessing linearity.

True volume	Replication 1	Replication 2	Replication 3	Replication 4
0.2	0.197	0.414	0.119	0.113
0.3	0.453	0.290	0.491	0.482
1.0	0.942	0.981	0.964	1.098
2.0	2.064	2.110	1.956	1.828
3.0	3.183	3.005	3.046	3.019
3.5	3.546	3.559	3.687	3.578
4.0	3.952	3.818	3.914	4.090
4.5	4.523	4.778	4.434	4.538
5.0	5.106	5.053	5.092	5.102

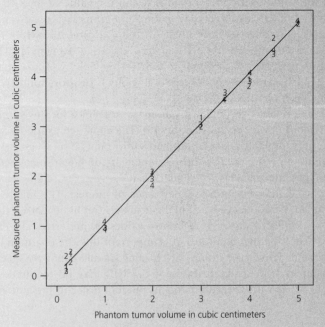

Figure 10.2 Illustration of concept of linearity.

Table 10.3 Results from fitting regression models.

	Estimate	Standard error	t-value	p-value
Linear model				
Intercept	0.0367	0.0330	1.1124	0.27
Volume	1.0022	0.0106	94.6628	<0.001
Curvilinear model				
Intercept	0.0654	0.0429	1.5268	0.14
Volume	0.9578	0.0436	21.9766	<0.001
Volume^2	0.0089	0.0085	1.0484	0.30
S-shaped model				
Intercept	0.0752	0.0570	1.3183	0.20
Volume	0.9282	0.1204	7.7084	<0.001
Volume^2	0.0234	0.0555	0.4225	0.68
Volume^3	−0.0018	0.0070	−0.2646	0.79

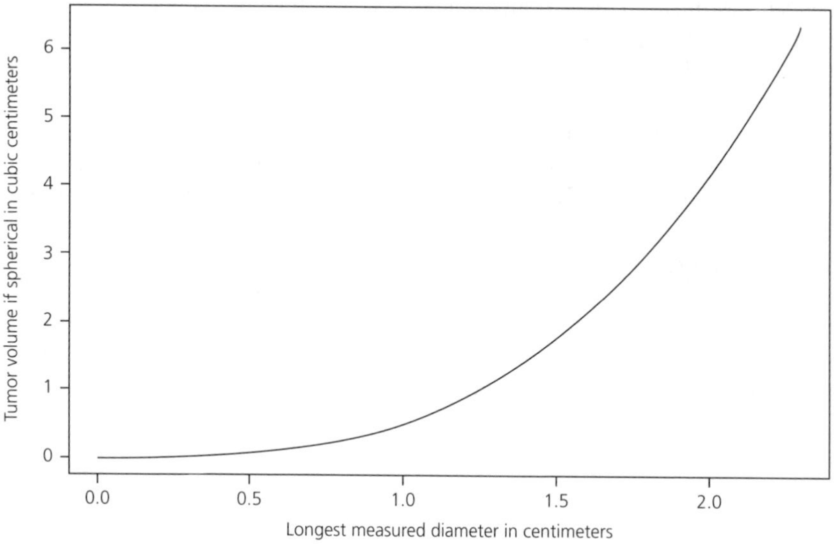

Figure 10.3 Illustration of nonlinear relationship between tumor diameter and volume.

Sometimes the value of the QIB is strictly increasing or decreasing in relationship to the value of the measurand, X, so that each value of X is associated with a unique value of Y, but this relationship is not linear. If we know the form of the relationship, we can apply a mathematical transformation to make it linear. An example of this would be the relationship between the volume of a spherical tumor and its diameter: $\text{volume} = \left(\pi \times \text{diameter}^3 \right) / 6$, shown in Figure 10.3.

Tumors that are close to spherical will have volumes that vary somewhat from this relationship to the longest measured diameter, whereas the relationship will not predict well the volumes of tumors that are elongated and/or flattened.

Commutability occurs "when the reference material reflects the *routine samples* (e.g. physical lesions in patients being imaged). It is what allows us to say that if a machine can measure tumor volume on a phantom with some precision and lack of bias, measurements of tumor volumes made on that same machine using a corresponding measurement procedure have the same precision and lack of bias for physical lesions in patients" [4]. This property of commutability is what we seek when constructing anatomical phantoms, which reflect the background noise against which the tumor signal must be detected and appropriately measured. It is more closely attained with specimens in which known values of the QIB are inserted, but such testing should be reserved for situations in which good measurement properties have already been shown in phantoms, so as not to waste tissue.

10.3.3 Measuring (analytical) precision

In the analytical context, **precision** is the "closeness of agreement between independent test/measurement results obtained under stipulated conditions." We will continue adapting procedures for laboratory assays, guided by CLSI EP5-A2 [10]. Definitions and procedures for the preclinical context are presented in Section 10.3.2.

As with earlier evaluations of technical properties in Section 10.2, we want to perform an experiment that incorporates factors that are known or strongly suspected to influence precision. These include day (at least 20), time of day (e.g., morning, afternoon; at least 2), tested measurand (e.g., phantom lesion; at least 2 per volume), and level of measurand (e.g., volume of phantom lesion; at least 2). Statistical analysis should use methods to correctly adjust for repeated observations. All quality control procedures, including calibration, should be used during the evaluation. The phantom used should adequately represent the organ in which we seek to make measurements. We will want to examine precision for a large measurand, a small measurand, and a measurand near a clinical decision point.

Example, continued

We will measure precision on 20 days, once in the morning and once in the afternoon at least 2 h later, for six spherical phantom lesions: two each at 0.5, 2, and 5 cm³. For each of these 40 measurement occasions, lesions will be measured in a random order. We analyze repeatability at each volume; here we will illustrate for 2 cm³. Let y_{ij1} be the measured volume of one of the 2 cm³ lesions in the morning run ($j=1$) or afternoon run ($j=2$) on day i for $i=1, ..., 20$ and y_{ij2} be the measured volume of the other 2 cm³ lesion (Table 10.4). Repeatability at 2 cm³ is then estimated as

$$S_r = \sqrt{\sum_{i=1}^{I}\sum_{j=1}^{2}\frac{\left(y_{ij1}-y_{ij2}\right)^2}{(4I)}}$$

for total number of days $I=20$. To estimate within-device precision at $2\,cm^3$, S_r, we will also estimate between-run SD, S_{rr}, and between-day SD, S_{dd}. Then $S_T = \sqrt{S_{dd}^2 + S_{rr}^2 + S_r^2} = 0.064$. This formula properly weighs the different contributors to variation, which pooling all of the measurements and taking an average do not (the SD will be too small). We can then calculate the coefficient of variation as $100\% \times S_r/2\,cm^3 = 3.2\%$.

Table 10.4 Estimating analytical precision.

Day	Morning 1	Morning 2	Afternoon 1	Afternoon 2	Morning mean	Afternoon mean	Daily mean
1	2.004	1.996	2.000	1.992	2.0000	1.9960	1.99800
2	1.999	2.019	2.000	2.025	2.0090	2.0125	2.01075
3	1.909	1.917	1.911	1.916	1.9130	1.9135	1.91325
4	1.984	1.983	2.042	2.039	1.9835	2.0405	2.01200
5	2.002	2.027	2.093	2.094	2.0145	2.0935	2.05400
6	2.045	2.041	2.023	2.019	2.0430	2.0210	2.03200
7	1.941	1.941	1.892	1.931	1.9410	1.9115	1.92625
8	2.069	2.082	2.018	2.032	2.0755	2.0250	2.05025
9	1.993	1.967	1.975	2.019	1.9800	1.9970	1.98850
10	1.888	1.885	1.844	1.832	1.8865	1.8380	1.86225
11	1.959	1.959	1.999	2.005	1.9590	2.0020	1.98050
12	2.081	2.082	2.026	2.029	2.0815	2.0275	2.05450
13	1.965	1.972	1.977	1.969	1.9685	1.9730	1.97075
14	2.133	2.126	2.119	2.126	2.1295	2.1225	2.12600
15	2.044	2.055	2.089	2.099	2.0495	2.0940	2.07175
16	1.987	1.99	1.97	1.98	1.9885	1.9750	1.98175
17	1.946	1.933	1.953	1.955	1.9395	1.9540	1.94675
18	1.932	1.956	1.951	1.966	1.9440	1.9585	1.95125
19	1.998	1.993	2.006	2.039	1.9955	2.0225	2.00900
20	1.961	1.967	2.024	2.025	1.9640	2.0245	1.99425

Sum of squared differences for morning = 0.003059.
Sum of squared differences for afternoon = 0.006214.
S_r = square root of $[(0.003059+0.006214)/(4\times20)] = 0.0062$.
Sum of squared differences between morning and afternoon = 0.027871.
A = square root of $[0.027871/(2\times20)] = 0.0264$. B = SD of daily mean = 0.0605.
$S_{dd}^2 = B^2 - \left(A^2/2\right) = 0.003308$. $S_{rr}^2 = A^2 - \left(S_r^2/2\right) = 0.000678$.
S_T = square root of $\left(S_{dd}^2 + S_{rr}^2 + S_r^2\_r\right) = 0.0634$. %CV = 3.2%.

10.3.4 Measuring change

An important use of a biomarker is to measure change over time—for example, monitoring tumor size or physiological activity during chemotherapy. This is reasonable when the measurand is at or above the LoQ, such that measured values have required precision to be clinically meaningful. We begin by defining "change"—Is it absolute, or relative? If we are interested in relative change, we must also define what it is relative to, for example, baseline. Next, we must state whether we are interested in any change—an increase or a decrease—or only in change in one of those directions. In order to determine whether a measured change is real, we need to know about the distribution of change measurements, including the precision with which change is measured. Finally, we consider how often we are willing to say that change has occurred if it really has not ("type I error rate") and how often we are willing to say that no change has occurred if it really has ("type II error rate") (see Chapter 8 for these definitions). These are each often set at 5%.

What about minimal detectable true change? Based on the previous text, we add 1.6, 1.7, 2.3, and 2.4 cm³ phantom lesions to our experiment, thinking carefully about time between measuring these and measuring the 2 cm³ phantom lesion. Again, we will assume that change values follow a normal distribution. When change is −0.4 cm³, measured values have mean = −0.404 and SD = 0.105, such that 95% of values lie below mean + 1.645 SD = −0.231; we would call these real change (Figure 10.4). When change is −0.3 cm³, measured values have mean = −0.302 and SD = 0.104, such that 95% of values lie below −0.131; we would not call these real change. A similar conclusion is drawn when change is 0.3 cm³ (Figure 10.4). When change is 0.4 cm³, measured values have mean = 0.408 and SD = 0.101, such that 95% of values lie above mean − 1.645 SD = 0.242, which we would call real change. If we measure change as outside ±0.2 cm³, we consider it to represent real change, based on the previous text. What we learn in this second experiment is that we can be comfortable that changes of ±0.4 cm³ will give us measured values outside ±0.2 cm³, in the appropriate direction.

Similar experiments should be performed for other baseline tumor volumes to gain insight into whether precision of measuring change is influenced by the size of the tumor at baseline.

10.3.5 Special situations: no meaningful zero and/or no ground truth

As we move closer to clinical measurements, we will encounter two special situations. The first is when there is no meaningful zero. We saw this with temperature: 0 degrees does not correspond to absence of temperature in the same way that 0 tumor volume corresponds to absence of tumor. Clinically, we might see this with functional imaging such as MRI diffusion coefficients and PET uptake values. In these situations ratios must be interpreted with extreme caution.

Example, continued

Before moving into the clinical context, we can learn about measuring change in our anatomical phantom. We will measure absolute change, in either direction. First, we will consider a situation of no change. We can perform an experiment similar to the analytical precision experiment, increasing complexity by adding different people into the design; this allows us to learn about what happens when, for example, two different technicians image the patient and baseline and follow-up. The analysis will be slightly more complex as well, to accurately reflect the experimental design. Let us take the result as showing that no change in a $2\,cm^3$ phantom lesion was measured with mean $= -0.003\,cm^3$ and SD $= 0.1\,cm^3$. If we assume that the change values follow a normal distribution, 95% of the values when no change occurs will lie within mean ± 1.96 SD $= (-0.199, 0.193)$ (Figure 10.4). We can then say that we are willing to consider change values outside of this interval as representing real change in tumor volume when baseline volume is $2\,cm^3$.

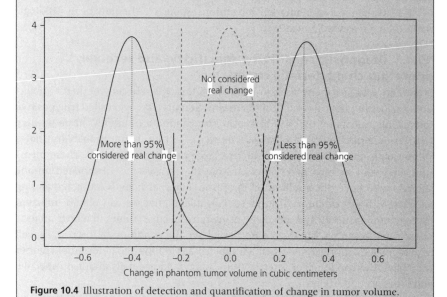

Figure 10.4 Illustration of detection and quantification of change in tumor volume.

The second situation is no ground truth. This is generally the situation when imaging a living patient—the measurand exists and has a true value; we just cannot obtain that value *in vivo*. It also applies to some extent when imaging tissue samples—for example, the size of a mass in excised tumor when imaged may be different from its size in the pathology lab. Without ground truth, we cannot measure bias. We then work instead with combined measures of precision.

Although it is tempting to use another measure based on its close agreement with truth in prior studies, this can produce assessments of the QIB's measurement properties that are not valid [6]. Specialized methods can be applied to situations when an imperfect reference standard is available or even, under several assumptions, when none is available [6]. These special methods may be used in addition to simple methods that seek to estimate variability without partitioning out components into systematic (bias) and random portions.

10.4 Evaluating clinical properties of QIBs

Consider ^{18}F-FDG uptake in Case example 1.2, (Chapter 1). Let us place ourselves at a point in research time where measurement of uptake can be achieved with very good analytical and preclinical properties. Evaluating the clinical properties of ^{18}F-FDG uptake as a biomarker for tumor response to the new drug, "Biologic A," is then a reasonable next step.

10.4.1 Diagnosis: sensitivity, specificity, and receiver operating characteristic curves

Sensitivity and specificity measure how well the QIB reflects whether a subject does or does not have a condition of interest. **Sensitivity**, also called true positive rate, is the probability that a subject with the condition of interest has a positive QIB result. **Specificity**, also called true negative rate, is the probability that a subject without the condition of interest has a negative QIB result. These measures were also defined in Chapter 9. Note that sensitivity is estimated among subjects who have the condition of interest, while specificity is estimated among subjects without condition of interest. This means that we can obtain unbiased estimates of sensitivity and specificity using retrospective studies in which subjects are selected based on whether or not they have the condition of interest, as well as prospective cohort studies in which subjects are followed to determine whether they have the condition of interest (see Chapter 7 for details about prospective and retrospective studies).

In Figure 10.5, eight subjects have the condition of interest and six of them test positive, for $Sens = 6/8 = 0.75$. Similarly, 16 subjects do not have the condition of interest and 13 do not test positive, for $Spec = 13/16 = 0.8125$ and $FPR = 0.1875$.

We can begin by considering sensitivity and specificity for some cutoff value, c, in uptake (see Chapter 9). In our example, tumor response is the condition of interest, so ^{18}F-FDG uptake values lower than c would indicate a positive test ("response"), and uptake values of c or more would indicate a negative test ("lack of response"). Note that $Sens(c)$, how often uptake correctly indicates that a subject is a responder, will be estimated only within responders and $Spec(c)$, how often uptake correctly indicates that a subject is a nonresponder, will be estimated only within nonresponders. This means that we can obtain unbiased estimates of $Sens(c)$ and $Spec(c)$ using case–control studies in which subjects are selected based

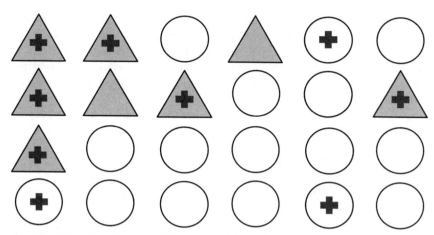

Figure 10.5 Hypothetical sample of 24 subjects, eight with the condition of interest (filled triangles) and 16 without the condition of interest (open circles). Subjects with positive QIB test results are indicated with a plus symbol.

on whether or not they are responders to Biologic A, as well as prospective cohort studies in which subjects are followed to determine whether they respond to Biologic A. The benefit of case–control studies is that they can be more efficient than cohort studies for this purpose.

The receiver operating characteristic (ROC) curve illustrates the trade-off in $Sens(c)$ and $Spec(c)$ as the cutoff c varies (see Chapter 9). The ROC curve plots the false-positive rate (FPR), obtained as $FPR(c) = 1 - Spec(c)$, on the x-axis, and $Sens(c)$ on the y-axis. In our example, $FPR(c)$ is the probability that a nonresponder has a positive QIB result, that is, an ^{18}F-FDG uptake value lower than c. If ^{18}F-FDG uptake value is a useless biomarker for tumor response, it will have the same probability of being positive whether or not the subject is a responder, that is, $Sens(c) = FPR(c)$. Another way to think about this is that every patient, whether or not she or he is a responder, would be equally likely to get a positive QIB result. A perfect QIB would have $Sens(c) = 1$ and $Spec(c) = 1$, that is, $FPR(c) = 0$, for some value of c. Such a situation rarely (if ever) occurs; but plotting the ROC curve can show us if there exists some cutoff for which the sensitivity and specificity pair can be clinically meaningful.

10.4.2 Prediction: positive and negative predictive value

Positive and negative predictive values can measure how well ^{18}F-FDG uptake predicts whether a patient will be a responder to Biologic A (see Chapter 9). Like $Sens(c)$ and $Spec(c)$, $PPV(c)$ and $NPV(c)$ depend on the cutoff for a positive test; unlike them, $PPV(c)$ and $NPV(c)$ also depend on prevalence.

If ^{18}F-FDG uptake tells us nothing beyond the prevalence of responders in the population—in other words, $PPV =$ prevalence and $NPV = 1$ minus prevalence—then it is not a useful biomarker, because the QIB result does not change the estimated probability of being a responder. The usefulness of ^{18}F-FDG uptake as a biomarker increases as *PPV* increases over prevalence and *NPV* increases over 1 – prevalence. Predictive values for the hypothetical example in Figure 10.5 support its potential utility: positive predictive value = 0.6667 is twice the prevalence (8/24 = 0.3333), and negative predictive value = 0.8667 is larger than one minus the prevalence (0.6667).

Predictive values can be estimated from *Sens* and *Spec* using **Bayes' theorem** as follows:

$$PPV = \{\text{prevalence} \times Sens\} / \left[\{\text{prevalence} \times Sens\} + \{(1 - \text{prevalence}) \times FPR\} \right].$$

$$NPV = \{(1 - \text{prevalence}) \times Spec\} / \left[\{(1 - \text{prevalence}) \times Spec\} + \{\text{prevalence} \times (1 - Sens)\} \right].$$

This relationship between predictive values and sensitivity, specificity, and prevalence is extremely useful when a retrospective study is used to estimate sensitivity and specificity. In retrospective studies, the prevalence of the condition in the study sample is often not representative of the clinical population; it is often much higher than the clinical population. If one were to calculate *PPV* and *NPV* directly from a retrospective study, these estimates would depend on the sample prevalence and would be misleading. Using Bayes' theorem, however, one can estimate *PPV* and *NPV* using estimates of sensitivity and specificity from a retrospective study and using the prevalence rate of the condition in the clinical population.

10.4.3 Association with patient outcomes

In Case example 1.2, FDG uptake is being investigated as a biomarker for recurrence of breast cancer. The goal is to assess the ability of FDG uptake, measured early in the course of treatment, to predict patient outcome. Here, the patient outcome of interest might be progression-free survival (PFS), breast cancer-specific mortality, or overall mortality. The QIB is the change in SUV_{max} over two time points following treatment.

There are two questions to address: (i) What is the accuracy of change in FDG uptake for predicting outcome? (ii) What is the difference in life expectancy for subjects with little change in FDG uptake versus subjects with reduced uptake?

For the first question we want to assess the accuracy of the change in FDG update for predicting outcome. In the early clinical assessment of a QIB, we don't know if the change between the baseline and the first treatment predicts recurrence or mortality or if the change between the baseline and the second treatment predicts outcome (or some other definition of change). We would want to use sensitivity, specificity, and/or ROC curves to determine if and when the change in FDG uptake predicts a future event.

Time-dependent ROC curves [11] are an important tool for assessing the accuracy of QIBs for clinical outcomes. This method takes into account that there is a time lag between the measurement of the biomarker (e.g., change in SUV) and the outcome (e.g., mortality), including the presence of censored data. ROC(t) describes the accuracy of a biomarker to predict events at time $t=t$.

A nice example of a study addressing the accuracy of a QIB is given in the study by Rousseau et al. [12]. After one course of a neoadjuvant chemotherapy, the sensitivity and specificity of the change in SUV since baseline were 61 and 96% for predicting pathologic response, and after the second treatment, they were 89 and 95%. The authors concluded that after two rounds of chemotherapy, FDG-PET accurately predicted pathologic response.

For the second question we want to compare the time until death (or time until recurrence) among subjects with negative QIB results (little change in FDG uptake over time) versus subjects with positive QIB results (reduced uptake). Such an analysis would require defining a cutpoint to group subjects as negative and positive. Often the median change in SUV_{max} at two early time points is used to group the subjects. This analysis seeks to determine whether metabolic responders live longer than nonresponders.

The statistical approach requires a comparison of survival curves, or time-to-event curves. The **Kaplan–Meier** (K-M) curve is the most commonly used; it illustrates the fraction of subjects living (or free of disease) for a certain amount of time. See Figures 4.2 and 4.5 for examples. This statistical method takes into account **censored data**, that is, the occurrence of subjects lost from the sample before the final outcome, that is, due to subject withdrawal from the study or the study ending before some subjects experience the study outcome. Censored data is common in long-term patient outcome studies. If censored observations are ignored or discarded in the analysis, the survival estimates from the study can be seriously biased. Thus, it is important to use statistical methods that account for censored data.

Particularly in nonrandomized studies, other important predictors of time to an event must be accounted, or adjusted, for in the analysis. An example would be including the subjects' age and gender in a time-to-event analysis where the event is death. **Cox proportional hazards regression** method is a modeling-based approach that can be used to adjust for important covariates, such as age, or to assess the effect of various predictors on survival times. Readers interested in more details about time-to-event analyses should see Klein and Moeschberger [13].

References

1 FDA, Drug Development Tools Qualifications Programs. 2014; Available from: http://www.fda.gov/Drugs/DevelopmentApprovalProcess/DrugDevelopmentToolsQualificationProgram/ucm284395.htm (accessed August 18, 2015).

2 Biomarkers Definitions Working Group, Biomarkers and surrogate endpoints: preferred definitions and conceptual framework. *Clin Pharmacol Ther*, 2001. **69**(3): p. 89–95.

3 Radiological Society of North America (RSNA), Quantitative Imaging Biomarkers Alliance. 2014; Available from: https://www.rsna.org/QIBA.aspx (accessed August 18, 2015).

4 Kessler, L.G., et al., The emerging science of quantitative imaging biomarkers terminology and definitions for scientific studies and regulatory submissions. *Stat Methods Med Res*, 2014.

5 Sickles, E., et al., ACR BI-RADS® Mammography, in *ACR BI-RADS® Atlas, Breast Imaging Reporting and Data System*, 2013, American College of Radiology: Reston, VA.

6 Obuchowski, N.A., et al., Quantitative imaging biomarkers: a review of statistical methods for computer algorithm comparisons. *Stat Methods Med Res*, 2015. **24**: p. 68–106.

7 Obuchowski, N.A., et al., Statistical issues in the comparison of quantitative imaging bio-marker algorithms using pulmonary nodule volume as an example. *Stat Methods Med Res*, 2015. **24**: p. 107–140.

8 CLSI EP17-A2, *Evaluation of Detection Capability for Clinical Laboratory Measurement Procedures; Approved Guideline—2nd ed.* 2012, CLSI: Wayne, PA.

9 CLSI EP6-A, *Evaluation of the Linearity of Quantitative Measurement Procedures; A Statistical Approach; Approved Guideline.* 2003, NCCLS: Wayne, PA.

10 CLSI EP5-A2, *Evaluation of Precision Performance of Quantitative Measurement Methods; Approved Guideline—2nd ed.* 2004, CLSI: Wayne, PA.

11 Heagerty, P.J., T. Lumley, and M.S. Pepe, Time-dependent ROC curves for censored survival data and a diagnostic marker. *Biometrics*, 2000. **56**(2): p. 337–344.

12 Rousseau, C., et al., Monitoring of early response to neoadjuvant chemotherapy in stage II and III breast cancer by [18F]fluorodeoxyglucose positron emission tomography. *J Clin Oncol*, 2006. **24**(34): p. 5366–5372.

13 Klein J.P. and M.L. Moeschberger, *Techniques for Censored and Truncated Data (Statistics for Biology and Health).* 2005, Springer: New York.

CHAPTER 11

Introduction to cost-effectiveness analysis in clinical trials

Ruth C. Carlos[1] and G. Scott Gazelle[2]

[1] University of Michigan Institute for Health Policy and Innovation and the Program for Imaging Comparative Effectiveness and Health Services Research, Ann Arbor, MI, USA
[2] Massachusetts General Hospital & Harvard Medical School, Boston, MA, USA

KEY POINTS

- Cost-effectiveness analyses represent a generic approach accounting for multiple potentially beneficial healthcare options, each option requiring resources to implement. Comparison between these options is expressed as the incremental cost per additional unit of health, usually a quality-adjusted life year.

- Comparative effectiveness research, explicitly comparing clinical effectiveness of competing health technologies or care strategies, coupled with cost-effectiveness analyses, allows comparison of relative value of disparate care options such as immunizations and cancer screening, permitting more informed decisions about resource allocation at the policy level.

- Generic health status instruments measure global health-related quality of life across populations and diseases and can be used to indirectly measure utilities used to determine a quality-adjusted life year. Choice of generic instrument to measure utilities can influence whether an intervention is deemed cost-effective.

- Disease-specific measures emphasize aspects of health status specific to a population, a disease, or a treatment.

- Choice of quality of life measures depends on the study goal; the domains of health important to the population, disease, or treatment; and the logistics of measure administration.

11.1 Introduction

The United States spent almost twice as much as per capita on healthcare compared to Norway, the next highest spending country in 2009 [1]. Our ability to pay for healthcare is outpaced by the rate of development of innovative healthcare

---

Handbook for Clinical Trials of Imaging and Image-Guided Interventions, First Edition.
Edited by Nancy A. Obuchowski and G. Scott Gazelle.

products and services. Further, the cost of care is increasingly shifted toward the insured, whose share of insurance premiums has increased three times as much as their earnings between 1999 and 2012 and has outstripped inflation over the same period [2].

It is *not* possible to provide *all* beneficial health services to *all* people. Implicit in that statement is the concept of rationing. Within our existing healthcare system, federal and state governments, managed care and accountable care organizations, employers, providers, and even private citizens and patients all ration or allocate healthcare resources.

Governments act as payers, deciding to expand public insurance schemes such as Medicaid to increase coverage and access to care as well as deciding which services will be covered. For example, most recently and most publicly, the government through Medicare has elected to cover lung cancer screening for high-risk smokers and former smokers [2, 3]. The federal government also acts as a provider, through the Veterans Affairs (VA) Medical Centers, restricting access to care to those whose benefits include access to VA services and determining which specific services are available to eligible individuals. Finally, the governments act as public health agencies, providing access to state-run childhood vaccination programs.

Managed care and accountable care organizations allocate health resources through benefit and health service coordination and predetermined healthcare networks for a fixed per capita payment or per care episode payment. Employers allocate health resources by acting as benefits managers selecting the health plans available for their employees. Providers allocate health resources in myriad ways at the hospital, physician group, and individual physician levels, for example, investing in one technology over another, providing only those services that are covered by the patients' insurance, and using a predetermined drug formulary. Even private citizens and patients allocate health resources, for example, delaying care to avoid a large cost share, accelerating the use of health services after the annual deductible has been met, and choosing to receive care from in-network providers even if out-of-network providers may be preferred. Most of these allocation decisions are not explicit, with a formal accounting of the costs and benefits.

In order to make rational decisions regarding the allocation of healthcare resources (i.e., rationing decisions), particularly at the societal level, explicit economic evaluation needs to be conducted, comparing alternative courses of action or care accounting for both the cost of care and the health consequences. The overarching goal is to achieve maximum value for each healthcare dollar spent, which in turn may be achieved either through lowering the cost of care or increasing patient benefit or both.

There are three general types of economic analyses that can be employed in healthcare evaluation: cost-minimization, cost–benefit, and cost-effectiveness analyses [4]; however, of these, cost-minimization and cost-effectiveness are most appropriate, depending on the circumstances.

11.2 Types of economic analyses

11.2.1 Cost-effectiveness analysis

Cost-effectiveness analysis (CEA) solves a generic problem where there are multiple potentially beneficial options, each option requiring resources to implement. Where resources are limited, as in healthcare, the overall goal is to optimize resource allocation. CEA accounts for the cost of care and the health benefits for competing strategies of care, the results of which are represented as the:

$$\frac{\text{Net change in resource cost}}{\text{Net change in health outcome (or effectiveness)}}$$

The result is interpreted as the **incremental cost-effectiveness ratio** (ICER) of the care strategy under investigation compared to the alternatives. ICER is expressed as dollars (or other monetary units) per additional health outcome, typically an additional year of life [4] or **quality-adjusted life year** (QALY).

Because CEA is a comparative analysis, the care strategy of interest and all its possible alternatives need to be considered at the outset. In these studies, doing nothing is an alternative that must generally be considered. This alternative incorporates the natural history of the disease and provides an effectiveness "floor" against which other strategies are evaluated. As an example, in a screening study, alternatives considered might include no screening, screening all individuals, or screening only certain high-risk individuals.

Resource costs must capture all the costs of providing the service, direct medical costs including hospitalizations, procedures, diagnostic tests, physician services, and miscellaneous supplies [5]. In addition, induced costs (and savings) that result from the intervention and any additional follow-up should be included in the analysis. In our screening example, induced costs related to a screening program might include the cost of managing a false-positive finding or the cost of treating a detected. The model should also account for nonmedical costs, such as time costs experienced by the patient, family, and caregiver and the cost of replacing activities that the patient can no longer perform (e.g., childcare).

Measures of health outcome or effectiveness include mortality (lives saved), morbidity (disabilities prevented), life years, QALYs, and disability-adjusted life years (DALYs) [6, 7]. The derivation of QALYs and the impact on cost-effectiveness will be discussed in the section on generic instruments for measurement of quality of life. Common measures of effectiveness are essential if one is to compare the results from different CEAs. In recent years, QALYs have become the preferred unit for effectiveness.

Because costs (and savings) accrue differently and the values placed on health outcomes vary to different stakeholders (society, health system, provider), the analytic perspective needs to be explicitly stated prior to conducting the analysis. The analytic perspective determines which costs are included in the model. Most

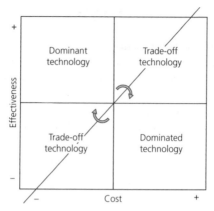

Figure 11.1 Results of a CEA mapped onto a four-quadrant space.

commonly, a societal or quasisocietal perspective is used in analyses that are intended to guide practice and policy. When conducted from a societal perspective, the model will include all costs regardless of who pays.

The results of a CEA (net cost/net benefit) can be mapped onto a four-quadrant space with cost at the *x*-axis and effectiveness at the *y*-axis (Figure 11.1) [8]. At the upper left quadrant, the care strategy under evaluation both costs less and yields more health benefits compared to the alternative and represents a "dominant" technology. Conversely, in the lower right quadrant, the care strategy costs more and yields fewer health benefits, thus representing a "dominated" technology. In the remaining quadrants, the care strategy either costs more with more benefits or cost less with fewer benefits compared to the alternative. In these spaces, trade-offs between cost and outcome can occur for cost-effective technologies. The definition of a cost-effective intervention is somewhat vague and depends on the willingness and ability of a society or population subgroup to pay for healthcare programs. Initially, programs with ICERs ≤ $60,000/QALY were considered "cost-effective." This threshold was initially derived from the cost of 1 year of dialysis care in the 1980s [9, 10], which was a service that was mandated to be covered in the United States. More recently, investigators have used $75,000–$100,000/QALY as a threshold for "cost-effectiveness." Of note, the National Institute for Clinical Excellence (NICE) in the United Kingdom has set 30,000 pounds/QALY as the threshold for coverage. However, there is no clear and commonly agreed-upon cutoff, and any threshold is probably best used as a guideline rather than an absolute.

11.2.2 Cost–benefit analysis

Cost–benefit analysis accounts for both the cost of care and the health consequence of care, where both the cost and the consequence are expressed in monetary units, rather than units of health. In healthcare, this type of analysis is not commonly conducted, perhaps due to the explicit valuation of a year of life in monetary terms, rather than the implicit valuation in a CEA.

11.2.3 Cost-minimization analysis

Cost-minimization analysis accounts for the cost of care when alternative care options have—or can be presumed to have—the same effectiveness. Before this type of analysis is undertaken, the medical evidence should be rigorously evaluated to ensure that the relevant health benefits are truly clinically equivalent [11]. Therefore, the strength of clinical evidence used to justify a cost-minimization analysis is critical to the reliability of the analysis, preferably using equivalence and noninferiority trials, rather than superiority trials. Cost-minimization analyses can be useful in comparing generic drugs with proprietary or name brands, where therapeutic equivalence is expected.

11.2.4 CEAs as part of comparative effectiveness research

Comparative effectiveness research (CER) is meant to explicitly compare the clinical effectiveness of competing technologies or care strategies, among the crowded field of technologies and strategies. CER by itself does not address the rising cost of care. CEA allows explicit evaluation of the relative value of one technology over another, even if the technologies address different diseases, for example, the cost-effectiveness of lung cancer screening by low-dose CT compared to living renal donor transplantation. This comparison of relative value permits stakeholders to potentially select from a "menu" of interventions and therefore make more informed decisions governing resource allocation, particularly at the policy level.

11.2.5 Summary

This overview summarizes the elements of different types of economic analyses with an emphasis on CEA. For in-depth discussion on the conduct of CEA including model building, additional resources are available [7]. Despite the limitations of CEA, it remains a useful analytical method that can be used to help guide the allocation of healthcare resources. However, at least in the United States, most would argue that the results of a CEA should be used in combination with other considerations in determining which healthcare services to provide.

11.3 Defining health-related quality of life

UNESCO defines quality of life as the "level of well-being of the society and the degree of satisfaction of a number of human needs" [12]. The term "well-being" has also been used to describe quality of life [13]. Rice refers to quality of life as the degree to which specified standards of living are met by objectively verifiable conditions, activities, and activity consequences of an individual's life [14]. All of these definitions encompass the totality of one's daily activities including the contribution of such diverse activities as social interaction with family and friends, job conditions, and even one's daily commute, which exercise an enormous impact on one's sense of well-being.

Health-related quality of life (HRQOL) refers to a smaller subset of components that impact health. The World Health Organization defines health as "a state of physical, mental and social well-being not merely the absence of disease or infirmity" [15]. HRQOL focuses on the impact of disease, disability, and disorder on one's well-being, including the change in one's well-being after resolution of disease, mitigation of disability, and reduction of disorder. Constituents of HRQOL include functional status, emotional status, symptoms, and global health.

11.3.1 Why measure HRQOL?

HRQOL measures the impact of disease on an individual patient or groups of patients. Imagine two individuals, Ray and Jean, both of whom awoke with a temperature of 100.8°F and wheezing. At an urgent care clinic, both had the same numerical elevations in white blood cell count and sedimentation rate and are diagnosed with a viral upper respiratory tract infection. Both take the same type and amount of analgesic and antipyretic. Ray returns home to bed for the rest of the day. Jean goes on to work a full day. Physiologic measures such as temperature and white blood cell count often correlate poorly with functional capacity and well-being. HQROL measures the variability of response to the same clinical condition, allowing us to understand the range of decrement to physical function and other constituents of HRQOL.

Measuring HRQOL allows an understanding of individual patient preferences to inform evidence-based medicine and decision-making. The US Preventive Services Task Force has recommended shared decision-making for diverse medical services as initiation of screening mammography in a 40-year-old woman [16] to aspirin chemoprevention for cardiovascular events in high-risk individuals [17]. In shared decision-making encounters, patient preferences for the service including the potential impact of the benefits and harms of the service on one's HRQOL contribute to the provider's recommendation for service initiation. Understanding patient preferences and values for the HRQOL impact of a disease versus an adverse event associated with disease prevention or treatment is particularly useful when there is no evidence supporting better outcomes with one treatment or another, when there is uncertainty out the optimum choice, or where the difference between the harms and benefits of treatment may be small [18]. Examples include choosing between watchful waiting and immediate prostatectomy in men with low-risk prostate cancer or initiation of tamoxifen for breast cancer prophylaxis in women who are BRCA positive. Patient preference may decide.

At a population level, assessment of cost-effectiveness of tests and interventions relies on the measurement of HQROL. Intuitively, a year spent in perfect health is valued differently than a year spent with a chronic illness, no matter how well controlled the illness is or how high functioning the individual is with the illness. Measuring HRQOL of health states permits definition of the quantity and the quality of a year of life lived in a given health state, yielding a QALY. These

QALYs provide a consistent measure of the benefits gained from interventions to prevent, diagnose, and treat disease by combining HRQOL and survival. The QALY measurement allows comparison of the societal value of disparate interventions such as childhood vaccinations and genome-specific chemotherapies and decisions on resource allocation [19].

11.3.2 Language of HRQOL

As with all disciplines, there is a specific vocabulary employed in the measurement of HRQOL. Briefly, an item refers to a question or component of a multipart question. An instrument refers to the questionnaire or survey. A domain or dimension of HRQOL refers to a behavior or experience. In the domain of physical function, subdomains may include mobility or self-care [20]. In the domain of emotional function, subdomains may include depression or anxiety.

11.4 Hierarchy of HRQOL measures

The measures used to evaluate the HRQOL have developed from two disciplines or traditions. These measures can be organized into a hierarchy of measures for population health (see Figure 11.2). In the tradition of the social sciences, the emphasis is on capturing the complexity of the disease condition with an emphasis on explanatory and descriptive variables. At the base of this hierarchy are health indicators, themselves not measures of HRQOL, for example, exposure to secondhand smoke or obesity in the community. These health indicators however can contribute to HRQOL, for example, physical function among obese individuals or social function among asthmatics exposed to secondhand smoke, often disease-specific scales or instruments.

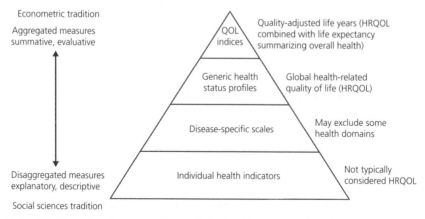

Figure 11.2 Hierarchy of measures for population health. Source: Adapted from Fryback [21]. © The National Academies.

11.4.1 Disease-specific instruments

Disease-specific instruments emphasize aspects of health status that are specific to the disease or treatment of interest. This may relate to a specific population, such as the adolescent or young adult cancer survivor who may be interested in HRQOL related to preservation of reproductive function, a specific disease such as osteoarthritis and the experience of pain, or to a specific physical or emotional function, such as sleep or depression. These measures assess disease severity or treatment progress in a patient or quantify the burden of disease in a population, focusing on the symptoms, functions, and emotions experienced by the patient population, but often exclude other domains of health that are not considered of interest. These instruments are constructed by developing questions or items that indicate specific aspects of the disease that are either empirically observed or theoretically derived. For example, the Functional Assessment of Cancer Therapy—Breast Cancer (FACT-B) provides a comprehensive evaluation of the domains of HRQOL experienced by patients treated for breast cancer including items related to physical function ("I am bothered by side effects of treatment") to sexual function after breast surgery ("I feel sexually attractive") and to postsurgical symptoms ("One or both of my arms are swollen or tender") [22]. These disease-specific scales are most commonly used in clinical trials of new therapeutic interventions. Because of their disease specificity, they are often difficult to administer to the general population.

11.4.2 Generic health status profiles

Generic health status profiles seek to assess the broad scope of HRQOL, measuring the domains important to all, using multiple subscales or subinstruments. For example, the EuroQOL-5D (EQ-5D) evaluates five domains: mobility, self-care, usual activities, pain/discomfort, and anxiety/depression [23, 24]. These can be used in a wide variety of settings, areas, diseases, and populations, allowing broad comparison of the relative impact of various healthcare programs such as mosquito control versus HIV medication versus organ transplantation. Because of the emphasis on global health, these measures may be insufficiently sensitive to changes in a specific condition or disease [20]. The most commonly used generic instruments will be reviewed and compared in a later section on selecting measures.

In the econometric tradition, there is emphasis on a single summary measure that expresses overall health as a function of quality combined with life expectancy. This "adjustment" for the health state reflects a patient's preference or utility for the treatment process and outcome. **Health utility measurement** is derived from economic and decision theory and is measured on a continuous scale from 0 (representing death) to 1 (representing perfect health), although a negative score representing health states worse than death are possible [25]. These scores represent both the health state and the value of the health state to the patient [20]. Utility measures for assessing the impact of treatment aggregate the positive effect of treatment efficacy and the negative effect of the treatment adverse events, without differentiating between the two. These measures are most useful in economic analyses comparing resource utilization and allocation to prioritize competing interventions, specifically CEAs. Utilities can be measured directly using the standard gamble or time-trade-off techniques [25]. Utilities can be measured indirectly from some generic instruments, specifically the EQ-5D and the Short Form-6D (SF-6D) using a scoring adjustment or index [20, 26], and are also termed HRQOL indices. These utilities are then multiplied by the estimated life expectancy to derive QALYs for a given disease or treatment.

QALY example: Patients with type 1 diabetes who have not been treated with dialysis nor renal transplantation were presented with hypothetical scenarios describing the health states of dialysis and of renal transplantation, derived from the Health Utilities Index descriptors [27]. Using a computer-aided standard gamble technique, patients valued the hypothetical state of dialysis at 0.70 and of renal transplantation at 0.80 (compared to perfect health at 1.0). Patients on dialysis have an average life expectancy of 7.82 years, rising to 18.30 years after living kidney transplantation. Therefore, quality-adjusted life expectancy on dialysis is 4.52 QALYs (0.70×7.82 years) and 10.29 QALYs after living kidney transplantation (0.80×18.30 years).

Considerations in measuring health utilities: In the previous OALY example, patients who have not yet experienced the health states being tested (viz., dialysis and renal transplantation) were being asked to estimate their hypothetical HRQOL. In this specific disease, the predicted HRQOL approximates the HRQOL experienced by those on hemodialysis and those who received renal transplantation [28]. In other diseases or treatments, prediction of quality of life after treatment is less reliable. For example, women scheduled for surgical treatment for breast cancer underestimate HRQOL associated with mastectomy compared to women who had been treated with mastectomy [29]. In a systematic review of utilities associated with dialysis, the standard gamble yielded the highest estimates and the SF-6D, the lowest [28] indicating that the method of utility elicitation yields different utility estimates, though the effect is not consistent across disease states. It is uncertain if these differences in utilities from elicitation techniques significantly impact CEAs.

11.4.3 What constitutes a "good" measure?

Before we discuss specific measures of HRQOL, it is useful to review the elements of a good measure. One can think of an HRQOL instrument as analogous to a diagnostic test requiring the same properties of a good test. As with a good test, a measure of HRQOL needs to be reliable, that is, reproducible both within patients (intraobserver reliability) and between patients (interobserver reliability). A measure also needs to be accurate, that is, validly captures the domains the instrument is meant to capture. Instrument reliability can be estimated by internal consistency, measured using Cronbach α coefficients. A larger coefficient indicates higher intercorrelation with the individual items in an instrument, in turn indirectly indicating the degree to which the instrument as a whole measures a single construct or domain of health [30–32]. A commonly accepted interpretation of

Table 11.1 Assessing instrument construct reliability.

Cronbach α coefficient	Internal consistency
$\alpha \geq 0.9$	Excellent
$0.7 \leq \alpha < 0.9$	Good
$0.6 \leq \alpha < 0.7$	Acceptable
$0.5 \leq \alpha < 0.6$	Poor
$0.5 < \alpha$	Unacceptable

instrument internal consistency using the Cronbach α coefficient is summarized in Table 11.1 [33]. These properties need to exist whether the instrument is evaluative or discriminative.

11.4.3.1 Evaluative instruments

Evaluative instruments measure the change in response within a patient or groups of patients over time [20]. The degree to which these measures are valid refers to the extent of correlation of change over time as predicted by a theoretical or conceptual model of disease or treatment. For example, the Brief Symptom Inventory was used to measure depression among individuals with multiple myeloma undergoing autologous stem cell transplantation. Measurement occurred at stem cell collection and again at 10 days after transplantation when toxicities are expected to be more intensive. As expected, anxiety and depression were higher on average at the later time point [34].

11.4.3.2 Discriminant instruments

Discriminant instruments measure the difference in response between patients or groups of patients at a specific point in time. The degree to which these measures are valid refers to the extent to which groups of patients with differing disease or treatment severity or outcomes can be differentiated. For example, HRQOL was measured in patients treated with trastuzumab, a monoclonal antibody directed at the human epidermal growth factor receptor (HER-2) in addition to chemotherapy compared to chemotherapy alone. The addition of trastuzumab to chemotherapy has previously been shown to prolong relapse-free and overall survival [35, 36]. Patients treated with the addition of trastuzumab experienced less fatigue, a higher physical function score, and greater global HRQOL as measured by the European Organization for Research and Treatment of Cancer Quality of Life Questionnaire [37].

The results of the instruments themselves must be interpretable to be clinically significant. Small, moderate, and large differences in measurements are expected to be correlated with small, moderate, and large degrees of clinical improvement or decline. A clinically significant change in HRQOL has been defined as a "difference score that is large enough to have an implication for the patient's treatment or care" [38]. This clinically significant difference from the perspective of the provider may be interpreted by the patient as the minimal important difference, the smallest change that remains meaningful to the patient experience, particularly salient in palliative rather than curative care. The clinical usefulness of studies reporting HRQOL depends on how accurately the study simulates the clinical experience, where HRQOL measured within a clinical trial with random assignment to treatment arms may not reflect actual clinical practice where patients have a choice of treatments. Disease-specific measures may be more relevant than global measures of health when discussing HRQOL, particularly in the context of shared decision-making [39, 40].

11.4.4 Generic measures

We will describe the two most commonly used generic measures used in the Cooperative Oncology Group trials, the SF-36 (and its variants) and the EQ-5D. In addition, we will describe the PROMIS-10, a generic measure developed by the NIH as part of its Toolbox across a range of ages, study designs, and settings to be incorporated into clinical trials.

The mostly used HRQOL generic measure is the *SF-36*, developed as a 36-question instrument derived from the much larger pool of questions used in the RAND Medical Outcomes Study (MOS) [22]. The purpose of the MOS was to develop practical tools for evaluating patient outcomes and to evaluate the impact of insurance, healthcare delivery system, clinician specialty training, and resource use intensity on those health outcomes [41]. The SF-36 has two main components: physical component scale (PCS) and the mental component scale (MCS). The PCS measures include physical function, pain, and role limitations due to physical health problems. The MCS measures include emotional well-being and role limitations due to emotional health problems. General health perceptions, vitality, and social function measures contribute to both the PCS and the MCS. All the component scales of the SF-36 have a good to excellent internal consistency (Cronbach $\alpha \geq 0.78$) [42], although reliability coefficients vary from 0.65 to 0.94 in demographic subgroups, disease type, and disease severity [22]. The SF-36 takes approximately 7–10 min to administer representing minimal burden on the respondent and the administrator. The SF-36 has subsequently been reduced to the SF-12 and the SF-6D. The PCS and MCS derived from SF-12, a 12-question instrument, are highly correlated with the PCS and MCS derived from the SF-36, when evaluated in a US population [43] and later replicated in a UK community sample and in a variety of UK patient groups including those with benign prostatic hypertrophy, Parkinson's disease, and congestive heart failure [44]. The SF-12 improves the efficiency and lowers the cost of administration at the price of fewer measurement levels and wider confidence intervals around PCS and MCS. The level of imprecision around the measurement estimate can be minimized with large group samples. The SF-6D represents a further reduction in the number of questions and domains of interest, using a six-dimensional health state classification (physical function, mental function, social function, general health perception, pain, and vitality) with 2–6 responses per domain, yielding a matrix of 9000 possible health states [45]. These health states have also been ranked by respondents to estimate patient preference or utility for these states using the standard gamble. Mapping the health states onto a utility measure allows transformation of a six-item instrument into a continuous scale that can then be used for CEAs. Further, both the SF-12 and SF-6D are proprietary instruments requiring licenses for use.

The **EuroQol Group** was a multicountry, multicenter, multidisciplinary group based in Europe to evaluate a standardized generic instrument of health with a key purpose of applicability to economic evaluation. The EQ-5D-5L measures five domains of health: mobility, self-care, usual activities, pain/discomfort, and anxiety/depression with five responses per domain yielding 3125 possible health states [23]. Similar to the SF-6D, the EQ-5D health states were ranked by respondents using the time-trade-off to allow measurement of patient preference or utility and transformation of the five-item instrument into a continuous scale to generate QALYs in CEAs. The EQ-5D is also proprietary.

The NIH has developed a series of nonproprietary open-access multidimensional measures assessing cognitive, emotional, motor, and sensory function for administration in patients aged 3–85 that can be applied across the broad range of diseases, study designs, and study settings, aggregated into the NIH Toolbox [46]. As part of this effort, the NIH has developed an extensive item bank of questions that measure patient-reported health status for physical, mental, and social well-being named the Patient-Reported Outcomes Measurement Information System (PROMIS) [47]. This effort includes development of both a global health instrument using 10 items (*PROMIS-10*) and a broad set of items that can be combined to measure domains of health specific to a range of diseases including cancer therapy, traumatic brain injury, and neurologic function. The global health instrument includes nine domains with excellent internal consistency reliability: self-rated health, physical health, mental health, overall quality of life, physical function, fatigue, emotional distress, and social health [48]. Determination of health utility from the PROMIS-10 was performed using regression analyses compared to the EQ-5D, rather than a comparison to preference measurement using the standard gamble or the time-trade-off [49]. Compared to the SF-36, the PROMIS-10 takes approximately 2 min to administer, similar to the SF-12 and the SF-6D. The PROMIS-10 is nonproprietary and does not require a license for use.

11.4.4.1 Comparison of generic measures
Table 11.2 compares the domains and content of the SF-6D, the EQ-5D-5L, and the PROMIS-10. Richardson et al. demonstrated a 0.116 absolute difference in utility measurements using the SF-6D and the EQ-5D-5L [50] measured in six countries across seven disease states from cancer to hearing loss to depression compared to the "healthy" population, with the SF-6D yielding lower utilities. Descriptive systems, that is, the domains of questions asked, how the questions are asked, and the number of questions within each domain, account for

Table 11.2 Comparison of the dimensions and content of three generic measures.

Dimension	SF-6D	EQ-5D-5L	PROMIS-10
Physical			
Physical ability/mobility/vitality/ coping/control	1*	1	1
Bodily function/self-care		1	
Pain/discomfort/fatigue	1	1	2
Usual activities/work	1	1	1
Psychosocial			
Depression/anxiety/anger	1	1	1
General satisfaction			1
Cognition/memory ability			1
Social function/relationships	1		1
(Family) role	1		
General quality of life			1
General health			1

Source: Adapted from Richardson [50].
*Number of items in each dimension.

approximately 77% of the difference. Scale effects, the use of different response scales for items in each of the instruments, account for the 3.5% of the difference in utilities. Micro-utility effects, the residual difference after accounting for descriptive systems and scale effects, represent approximately 20% of differences in utilities. In a US sample, comparison of EQ-5D-5L actual utilities to those predicted by PROMIS-10 demonstrated absolute differences between 0.01 and 0.03 [49]. Although the PROMIS-10 was not explicitly compared to the SF-6D and the EQ-5D-5L, it is likely that similar sources of differences in utility measures exist.

In a study conducted by the NCI Cancer Care Outcomes Research and Surveillance (CanCORS) Consortium comparing the EQ-5D and the SF-6D in newly diagnosed lung cancer patients, absolute differences in utilities of 0.10 were demonstrated with the SF-6D yielding lower utilities, similar to Tramontano [51]. The EQ-5D demonstrated a significant ceiling effect with 20% of patients rating their health as perfect, suggesting that the EQ-5D is relatively insensitive to small differences in health when the population is generally high functioning and is unlikely to capture health improvement in this population. The SF-6D had previously been demonstrated to have floor effects, with a large proportion of respondents reporting the most severe level of health possible. For example, in a large sample of liver transplant patients, 42% responded at the most severe level of role limitation domain [52]. Floor effects would limit the ability of the instrument to detect additional decrease in function in the affected domains in these patients. The EQ-5D does not suffer from similar floor effects.

These small differences in utility measurement may have significant impact on the assessed cost-effectiveness of interventions in a variety of settings such as end-stage renal disease [53], tumor necrosis factor inhibition in rheumatoid arthritis [54], and total disc replacement in low back pain [55], with less favorable cost-effectiveness of interventions when the SF-5D is used to adjust for QALYs.

11.4.4.2 Considerations in generic measure selection

There are only minimal differences in respondent and administration burden between the SF-6D, the EQ-5D, and the PROMIS-10. The SF-6D may be more useful in high-functioning or generally healthy patients due to the absence of a ceiling effect, while the EQ-5D is more appropriate in patients with worse health states due to the absence of a floor effect. The PROMIS-10 is nonproprietary without the need for license fees for use and may be appropriate in trials with nominal budgets. Regardless of the measure chosen, the investigator needs to be aware of the potential impact the utility measure used on assessed cost-effectiveness of an intervention.

11.4.5 Disease-specific measures

There are innumerable disease-specific measures developed and used within the literature, and it is beyond the scope of this review to evaluate even a significant proportion of the measures. For investigators interested in cancer measures, the Functional Assessment of Cancer Therapy series of instruments provide for a range of specific cancers (http://www.facit.org/FACITOrg/Questionnaires [21]. Accessed February 22, 2015). In addition to general health and well-being, disease-specific domains include concerns associated with cancer-specific treatments, for example, evaluating bowel-specific concerns in patients with colon cancer and swallowing in patients with head and neck cancer. Similarly, the MD Anderson Symptom Inventory (MDASI) uses a 13-item core with additional disease-specific modules (http://www.mdanderson.org/education-and-research/departments-programs-and-labs/departments-and-divisions/symptom-research/symptom-assessment-tools/mdanderson-symptom-inventory.html. Accessed February 22, 2015) [56]. The PROMIS instruments provide similar disease- and symptom-specific instruments (https://www.assessmentcenter.net/documents/InstrumentLibrary.pdf [57]. Accessed February 22, 2015). PROMIS has the added advantage of computerized adaptive testing administering a variable through parsimonious number of items to measure a domain of health as determined by the answer to the preceding question. This allows greater flexibility in administration and improved reliability particularly of longitudinal assessments.

11.4.5.1 Considerations in disease-specific measure selection: a case-based example

Selection of disease-specific measures can be complex and depends on the underlying clinical condition, the type of intervention being assessed, and the presumed impact of the intervention on HRQOL. As a working example, we will assess the selection of a disease-specific measure in knee pain interventions.

Table 11.3 Comparison of the dimensions and content of four knee pain-specific measures.

Domain	AKSS	WOMAC	HSS	OKS
Pain severity	1	5 (different activities)	2 (rest, walking)	2 (average, standing)
Pain medication	—	—	—	—
Pain quality	—	—	—	—
Temporality of pain	1 (occasional or continuous)	1 (at night)	—	1 (at night)
Physical function	1 (walk, stand)	4 (walk, climb, sit, stand)	1 (walk)	3 (normal work, distance before severe, stand)
Emotional function				2 (troubled at night, unbearable pain)

AKSS = American Knee Society Score.
WOMAC = Western Ontario and McMaster Universities Osteoarthritis Index.
HSS = Hospital for Special Surgery Knee Score.
OKS = Oxford Knee Score.
Source: Adapted from Wylde [58].

According to the Initiative on Methods, Measurement, and Pain Assessment in Clinical Trials (IMMPACT) consensus statement in chronic pain trials, measurement of the effect of an intervention should evaluate the multiple dimensions of pain including severity (e.g., average pain vs. worst pain), temporality (e.g., worst at night), quality (e.g., dull vs. sharp), and use of pain medication; multiple dimensions of function including physical and emotional function; and a global assessment of improvement.

Table 11.3 compares the domains and content of four common knee pain-specific HRQOL measures. Not all instruments measure pain temporality with only one measuring emotional function. None of the instruments measure pain quality or medication use. Ideally one would select the measure that covers the most domains of chronic pain, augmented with additional instruments measuring any omitted domains. If comparison to an existing study or existing intervention is desired, then the instrument selected should be comparable across both studies and interventions, supplemented by additional instruments if the one previously used had domain deficiencies. As a final consideration, one may choose what is commonly accepted as a reasonable instrument in one's area of study to achieve face validity of the study, again augmented with additional instruments for missing domains.

11.4.6 Other considerations in measure selection

Table 11.4 suggests a series of possible generic and disease-specific measures guided by the ultimate goal of the trial or study.

Other considerations in measure selection include consideration of the respondent who may be the patient himself or herself, a surrogate such as a parent or a

Table 11.4 Suggested HRQOL measures by study goal.

Study goal	Possible measures
Assess diagnostic imaging test or imaging-based treatment efficacy	Disease-specific measure, toxicity symptoms, global health, health utilities
Minimize disease symptoms	Disease-specific measure, toxicity symptoms, global health, functional status, health utilities
Cure disease	Survival, health utilities, toxicity symptoms, functional status
Palliate/prolong survival	Survival, functional status, disease-specific measure, global rating, health utilities
Characterize illness burden in a population	Generic health status profile
Characterize illness burden in a specific patient	Generic health status profile, domain-specific measures
Predict outcomes	Baseline HRQOL
CEA/CUA	Health utilities

caregiver, or the provider. Mode of administration should also be considered with in-person and phone administration yielding the most complete data at the highest cost. Other modes include mail or online self-administered [59].

11.4.7 Summary

Ultimately, there is no right or wrong choice of measure as long as the instrument choice is guided by the psychometric properties of the instrument that fits the population and disease of interest.

References

1 OECD (2014) Total expenditure on health per capita, Health: Key Tables from OECD, No. 2. Available from: http://dx.doi.org/10.1787/hlthxp-cap-table-2014-1-en (accessed September 18, 2015).

2 Claxton, G., et al., Health benefits in 2012: moderate premium increases for employer-sponsored plans; young adults gained coverage under ACA. *Health Aff (Millwood)*, 2012. **31**(10): p. 2324–2333.

3 Decision Memo for Screening for Lung Cancer with Low Dose Computed Tomography (LDCT) (CAG-00439N). Available from https://www.cms.gov/medicare-coverage-database/details/nca-decision-memo.aspx?NCAId=274 (accessed September 11, 2015).

4 Eisenberg, J.M., Clinical economics: a guide to the economic analysis of clinical practices. *JAMA*, 1989. **262**(20): p. 2879–2886.

5 Luce, B., et al., Estimating costs in cost-effectiveness analysis, in *Cost-Effectiveness in Health and Medicine: Report of the Panel on Cost-Effectiveness in Health and Medicine*, M.R. Gold, et al., Editors. 1996, Oxford University Press: New York, pp. 176–213.

6 Torrance, G.W. and D. Feeny, Utilities and quality-adjusted life years. *Int J Technol Assess Health Care*, 1989. **5**(04): p. 559–575.

7 Gold M.R, D.L. Patrick, and G.W. Torrance, Identifying and valuing outcomes, in *Cost-Effectiveness in Health and Medicine: Report of the Panel on Cost-Effectiveness in Health and Medicine*, M.R. Gold, J.E. Siegel, and L. Russel, Editors. 1996, Oxford University Press: New York.

8 Petrou, S. and A. Gray, Economic evaluation alongside randomised controlled trials: design, conduct, analysis, and reporting. *BMJ*, 2011. **342**: p. d1548.

9 Hirth, R.A., et al., Willingness to pay for a quality-adjusted life year: in search of a standard. *Med Decis Making*, 2000. **20**(3): p. 332–342.

10 Weinstein MC, From cost-effectiveness ratios to resource allocation: where to draw the line?, in *Valuing Health Care: Costs, Benefits, and Effectiveness of Pharmaceuticals and Other Medical Technologies*, F.A. Sloan, Editor. 1995, Cambridge University Press: New York.

11 Duenas, A., Cost-minimization analysis, in *Encyclopedia of Behavioral Medicine*. M. Gellman and J. Turner, Editors. 2013, Springer: New York. p. 516.

12 Quality of Life Improvement Programmes, *APPEAL Training Materials for Continuing Education, Vol IV*. 1993, UNESCO Principal Regional Office for Asia and the Pacific, Bangkok. p. 1.

13 Andrews, F. and A. McKennell, Measures of self-reported well-being: their affective, cognitive, and other components. *Soc. Indic. Res.*, 1980. **8**: p. 127–155.

14 Rice, R., Work and the quality of life, in *Applied Socially Psychology Annual. 5: Applications in Organizational Settings*, S. Oskamp, Editor. 1984, Sage: Beverly Hills, CA. p. 155–177.

15 Preamble to the Constitution of the World Health Organization as adopted by the International Health Conference, New York, 19–22 June, 1946; signed on 22 July 1946 by the representatives of 61 States. Available from http://www.who.int/governance/eb/who_constitution_en.pdf (accessed September 11, 2015).

16 U.S. Preventive Services Task Force, Screening for breast cancer: U.S. Preventive Services Task Force recommendation statement. *Ann Intern Med*, 2009. **151**(10): p. 716–726, w-236.

17 U.S. Preventive Services Task Force, Aspirin for the primary prevention of cardiovascular events: recommendation and rationale. *Ann Intern Med*, 2002. **136**(2): p. 157–160.

18 Sheridan, S.L., R.P. Harris, and S.H. Woolf, Shared decision making about screening and chemoprevention. a suggested approach from the U.S. Preventive Services Task Force. *Am J Prev Med*, 2004. **26**(1): p. 56–66.

19 Sassi, F., Calculating QALYs, comparing QALY and DALY calculations. *Health Policy Plan*, 2006. **21**(5): p. 402–408.

20 Guyatt, G.H., D.H. Feeny, and D.L. Patrick, Measuring health-related quality of life. *Ann Intern Med*, 1993. **118**(8): p. 622–629.

21 Fryback, D.G. (2010). *Measuring Health-Related Quality of Life*. Paper prepared for the Workshop on Advancing Social Science Theory: The Importance of Common Metrics. National Academies, Washington, DC, February 25–26.

22 FACIT.org, 2015; Available from: http://www.facit.org/FACITOrg/Questionnaires (accessed February 22, 2015).

23 Coons, S.J., et al., A comparative review of generic quality-of-life instruments. *Pharmacoeconomics*, 2000. **17**(1): p. 13–35.

24 Euroqol.org, 2015; Available from: http://www.euroqol.org/about-/how-to-use-eq-5d.html (accessed February 22, 2015).

25 Boyle, M.H., et al., Economic evaluation of neonatal intensive care of very-low-birth-weight infants. *N Engl J Med*, 1983. **308**(22): p. 1330–1337.

26 Bleichrodt, H. and M. Johannesson, Standard gamble, time trade-off and rating scale: experimental results on the ranking properties of QALYs. *J Health Econ*, 1997. **16**(2): p. 15–75.

27 Brazier, J., et al., A comparison of the EQ-5D and SF-6D across seven patient groups. *Health Econ*, 2004. **13**(9): p. 873–884.

28 Knoll, G.A. and G. Nichol, Dialysis, kidney transplantation, or pancreas transplantation for patients with diabetes mellitus and renal failure: a decision analysis of treatment options. *J Am Soc Nephrol*, 2003. **14**(2): p. 500–515.

29 Wyld, M., et al., A systematic review and meta-analysis of utility-based quality of life in chronic kidney disease treatments. *PLoS Med*, 2012. **9**(9): p. e1001307.

30 Waljee, J.F., et al., The choice for breast cancer surgery: can women accurately predict postoperative quality of life and disease-related stigma? *Ann Surg Oncol*, 2011. **18**(9): p. 2477–2482.

31 Cortina, J., What is coefficient alpha? An examination of theory and applications. *J Appl Psychol*, 1993. **78**(1): p. 98–104.

32 Schmitt, N., Uses and abuses of coefficient alpha. *Psychol Assess*, 1996. **8**: p. 350–353.

33 Zinbarg, R., et al., Estimating generalizability to a universe of indicators that all have an attribute in common: a comparison of estimators for alpha. *Appl Psychol Meas*, 2006. **30**: p. 121–144.

34 Kline, P., *Handbook of Psychological Testing*. 2013, Taylor & Francis, London.

35 Sherman, A.C., et al., Changes in quality-of-life and psychosocial adjustment among multiple myeloma patients treated with high-dose melphalan and autologous stem cell transplantation. *Biol Blood Marrow Transplant*, 2009. **15**(1): p. 12–20.

36 Cobleigh, M.A., et al., Multinational study of the efficacy and safety of humanized anti-HER2 monoclonal antibody in women who have HER2-overexpressing metastatic breast cancer that has progressed after chemotherapy for metastatic disease. *J Clin Oncol*, 1999. **17**(9): p. 2639–2648.

37 Slamon, D.J., et al., Use of chemotherapy plus a monoclonal antibody against HER2 for metastatic breast cancer that overexpresses HER2. *N Engl J Med*, 2001. **344**(11): p. 783–792.

38 Osoba, D., et al., Effects on quality of life of combined trastuzumab and chemotherapy in women with metastatic breast cancer. *J Clin Oncol*, 2002. **20**(14): p. 3106–3113.

39 Wyrwich, K.W., et al., Estimating clinically significant differences in quality of life outcomes. *Qual Life Res*, 2005. **14**(2): p. 285–295.

40 Guyatt, G.H., et al., Users' guides to the medical literature. XII. How to use articles about health-related quality of life. Evidence-Based Medicine Working Group. *JAMA*, 1997. **277**(15): p. 1232–1237.

41 Schunemann, H.J., E.A. Akl, and G.H. Guyatt, Interpreting the results of patient reported outcome measures in clinical trials: the clinician's perspective. *Health Qual Life Outcomes*, 2006. **4**: p. 62.

42 Stewart, A.L. and J.E. Ware, *Measuring Functioning and Well-Being: The Medical Outcomes Study Approach*. 1992, Duke University Press: Durham, NC.

43 Hays, R.D., C.D. Sherbourne, and R.M. Mazel, The RAND 36-Item Health Survey 1.0. *Health Econ*, 1993. **2**(3): p. 217–227.

44 Ware, J., Jr., M. Kosinski, and S.D. Keller, A 12-Item Short-Form Health Survey: construction of scales and preliminary tests of reliability and validity. *Med Care*, 1996. **34**(3): p. 220–233.

45 Jenkinson, C. and R. Layte, Development and testing of the UK SF-12 (short form health survey). *J Health Serv Res Policy*, 1997. **2**(1): p. 14–18.

46 Brazier, J., et al., Deriving a preference-based single index from the UK SF-36 Health Survey. *J Clin Epidemiol*, 1998. **51**(11): p. 1115–1128.

47 NIH Toolbox, For the Assessment of Neurological and Behavioral Function. 2015; Available from: http://www.nihtoolbox.org/Pages/default.aspx (accessed August 18, 2015).

48 Cella, D., et al., The Patient-Reported Outcomes Measurement Information System (PROMIS): progress of an NIH Roadmap cooperative group during its first two years. *Med Care*, 2007. **45**(5 Suppl 1): p. S3–S11.

49 Hays, R.D., et al., Development of physical and mental health summary scores from the patient-reported outcomes measurement information system (PROMIS) global items. *Qual Life Res*, 2009. **18**(7): p. 873–880.

50 Revicki, D.A., et al., Predicting EuroQol (EQ-5D) scores from the patient-reported outcomes measurement information system (PROMIS) global items and domain item banks in a United States sample. *Qual Life Res*, 2009. **18**(6): p. 783–791.

51 Richardson, J., A. Iezzi, and M.A. Khan, Why do multi-attribute utility instruments produce different utilities: the relative importance of the descriptive systems, scale and "micro-utility" effects. *Qual Life Res*, 2015. **24**(8): p. 2045–2053.

52 Tramontano, A.C., et al., Catalog and comparison of societal preferences (utilities) for lung cancer health states: results from the Cancer Care Outcomes Research and Surveillance (CanCORS) Study. *Med Decis Making*, 2015. **35**(3): p. 371–387.

53 Longworth, L. and S. Bryan, An empirical comparison of EQ-5D and SF-6D in liver transplant patients. *Health Econ*, 2003. **12**(12): p. 1061–1067.

54 Yang, F., et al., Comparison of the preference-based EQ-5D-5L and SF-6D in patients with end-stage renal disease (ESRD). *Eur J Health Econ*, 2014.

55 Kvamme, M.K., et al., Cost-effectiveness of TNF inhibitors vs synthetic disease-modifying antirheumatic drugs in patients with rheumatoid arthritis: a Markov model study based on two longitudinal observational studies. *Rheumatology (Oxford)*, 2015. **54**(7): p. 1226–1235.

56 Johnsen, L.G., et al., Cost-effectiveness of total disc replacement versus multidisciplinary rehabilitation in patients with chronic low back pain: a Norwegian multicenter RCT. *Spine (Phila Pa 1976)*, 2014. **39**(1): p. 23–32.

57 MD Anderson Cancer Center, The MD Anderson Symptom Inventory (MDASI). 2015; Available from: http://www.mdanderson.org/education-and-research/departments-programs-and-labs/departments-and-divisions/symptom-research/symptom-assessment-tools/mdanderson-symptom-inventory.html (accessed February 22, 2015).

58 The Assessment Center Instrument Library, Instruments Available for Use in Assessment Center. 2015; Available from: https://www.assessmentcenter.net/documents/InstrumentLibrary.pdf (accessed February 22, 2015).

59 Wylde, V., et al., Assessment of chronic postsurgical pain after knee replacement: a systematic review. *Arthritis Care Res (Hoboken)*, 2013. **65**(11): p. 1795–1803.

60 Gwaltney, C.J., A.L. Shields, and S. Shiffman, Equivalence of electronic and paper-and-pencil administration of patient-reported outcome measures: a meta-analytic review. *Value Health*, 2008. **11**(2): p. 322–333.

Index

Handbook for Clinical Trials of Imaging and Image-Guided Interventions, First Edition.
Edited by Nancy A. Obuchowski and G. Scott Gazelle.
© 2016 John Wiley & Sons, Inc. Published 2016 by John Wiley & Sons, Inc.